"Frances Jones's book, *Overcoming* _____ _____ *Barren but Not Ashamed*, is a blessing to women with infertility. The book details her personal experience with infertility; her faith, marriage, and journey of discovery; and how she overcame the emotional stigmas of infertility. After reading the book, I was amazed by how many life experiences we share. Frances not only encourages me as a woman with infertility, but she also encourages my faith. Her book provides emotional coping mechanisms, strategies, and steps on how to break free from tormenting thoughts, and teaches how to get your power back. It is a must-read for anyone who has experienced infertility. Make it part of your reference library."

—Shervonne Coney, Founder of Black Women and Infertility

"Infertility impacts one in eight couples, yet many suffer alone and in silence. Thank you, Frances Jones, for sharing your story to help increase awareness and shatter the stigmas that surround this issue. Your personal journey through physical and emotional struggles on your way to finding peace again is inspirational. Many will find comfort in this book."

—Lora Shahine, MD, FACOG, Director of Patient Experience and Outreach, Pacific NW Fertility, Clinical Assistant Professor University of Washington, and author of the best-selling *Not Broken: An Approachable Guide to Miscarriage and Recurrent Pregnancy Loss*

"Frances Jones's book, *Overcoming the Emotional Stigmas of Infertility: Barren but Not Ashamed*, describes perfectly the ongoing struggles facing those of us saddled with this traumatic, often isolating diagnosis. Though the physical pains and hassles are many, it is the emotional toil that incessantly sticks with patients. After miscarriages and multiple rounds of IVF, I have been blessed with three beautiful babies, but as I read through Frances's story, I was immediately transported back to those dark, emotional days of desperation. I admire her strength and determination as she pulled herself out of that darkness and chose to light the way with hope for others traveling this uncertain path."

—Danette Kubanda, Emmy Winning Television Producer, Publicity Consultant, Media Coach, Writer

"Frances Jones has a heart of pure gold. In her book, *Overcoming the Emotional Stigmas of Infertility: Barren but Not Ashamed*, Frances Jones openly shares her innermost thoughts, raw emotion, and how she overcame feelings of inadequacy, shame, and rejection brought on by infertility. In a world where many hide behind the mask of a smile, Frances boldly shares her testimony in the hope of comforting and equipping women with transformative tools to overcome, just as she did. If you have been suffering in silence, Frances' book will give you the keys you need by faith to regain your power and your purpose."

—Min. Nakita Davis, CEO and Founder of @jesuscoffeeandprayer

"Frances Jones's book, *Overcoming the Emotional Stigmas of Infertility: Barren but Not Ashamed*, is a must-read. Her life-changing story takes the reader on an empowering journey through her personal battle with infertility and the negative emotions she encountered along the way, and gives the reader renewed hope, faith, and self-worth. Anyone wanting to be free from the negative emotions and stigmas associated with infertility needs to read it and keep it in their reference library."

—Mollie Walker, Co-Founder of Tennessee Fertility Advocates

"Overcoming the Emotional Stigmas of Infertility: Barren but Not Ashamed is a must-read for anyone who has experienced infertility. By writing her story in an authentic and personal way, Frances Jones pulls open the curtain of the negative and self-destructive thoughts and feelings that often come with infertility but are rarely spoken. She will empower you to take charge of your internal dialogue, walking you toward emotional freedom from the scars borne from infertility. I will be adding this book to my recommended reading list for my Trying to Conceive (TTC) tribe."

—Kara Edwards, Founder, Starfish Infertility Foundation

"It is not easy to share intimate details of one's life, especially the stories that affect us deeply, but that is exactly what Frances Jones has done. As I read her story about her infertility journey, her words struck my heart deeply. I felt her sadness, bitterness, and negative energy. As you read *Overcoming the Emotional Stigmas of Infertility: Barren but Not Ashamed*, you will learn of the emotions that Frances experienced, her response to her dashed dreams and desires, and how she healed herself. I had no idea that my own thoughts toward baby showers and the negativity I had toward pregnant women were affecting me so much. As I read her advice and how she feels now, my heart began to soften. I knew that I wasn't alone and that someone else had been on the same journey. Her "Questions to Ponder" and the exercises she provides to gain peace showed how she healed her heart, and helped me to do the same."

—Laura Coleman, Accredited Financial Counselor
and Adoption Money Coach

Overcoming the Emotional Stigmas of Infertility

Overcoming the Emotional Stigmas of Infertility

Barren But Not Ashamed

Frances Jones, M.A

Foreword by William H. Kutteh, MD, PhD

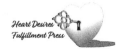

Heart Desires Fulfillment Press

Heart Desires Fulfillment Press
1138 N Germantown Pkwy
Ste 101-349
Cordova, TN 38016
855-738-5345
www.heartdesirescoaching.com

ISBN (paperback): 978-1-7356340-0-5
ISBN (ebook): 978-1-7356340-1-2

Printed in the United States of America

Edited by Jessica Vineyard, Red Letter Editing, www.redletterediting.com
Cover and interior design by Christy Collins, Constellation Book Services

Dedication

To my parents, the late Jeffrey and Lucille Rowell.

Contents

Acknowledgments

I would like to thank my husband and best friend, Christopher Jones, for the love, support, and confidence you have in me. You helped me find the courage and strength to share with people the painful part of my life that I have kept hidden for a very long time.

To my siblings, thank you for cheering me on, reviewing my chapters, and giving me encouraging feedback as I wrote.

To my three beautiful children and four adorable grandchildren, thank you for all of the fun memories you have given me. I can honestly say that the branches of my part of the family tree, which I never thought would have life, are growing stronger and more vibrant each day.

Thank you to my parents, Jeffrey and Lucille Rowell. The love, guidance, and teachings that you imparted into my heart will forever stay with me. I am eternally grateful for the sacrifices you made and the parental examples you gave. Not only did you give me life, you demonstrated one of the most important gifts of all, faith.

Special thanks to Martha Bullen, Debra Englander, Cristina Smith, my publishing team, and Raia King in marketing for your guidance, professional insight, and encouraging feedback. You gave me the confidence needed to make my book a reality. Thank you to Danette Kubanda for helping me to prepare for media presence. Thank you to my editor, Jessica Vineyard; book cover designer, Christy Collins; image consultant, Mary Giuseffi; and photographer, Alex Ginsburg, for your part in helping me to present my book in written and pictorial form. I am truly grateful for your assistance.

To every person who has been affected in some way with infertility, maybe you have been vocal about your fertility challenges or, like me, have kept them hidden from those around you. In either case, my message is simple: be encouraged. Hurting hearts can be healed.

Foreword

*O*vercoming *the Emotional Stigmas of Infertility: Barren but Not Ashamed* is a personal reflection of Frances Jones's twenty-year journey and a valuable life story of how one couple dealt with their fertility and infertility. Frances takes the reader from her childhood experiences in dealing with a large family through the personal challenges that she encountered in her desire to have children.

A small part of the book deals with the actual fertility treatments, the challenges that she had with her insurance company, and the care that she received by her multiple physicians. However, the main focus of the book, and the value to the reader, is in understanding the emotions that she went through and the feelings that she had during this time.

Frances takes the reader through periods of shame, embarrassment, and low self-esteem, and explains the tools she used to get out of this dark zone and move to where she could respect herself and her family. Ultimately, she was unable to have children of her own but had a large family through adoption.

Frances offers tips to couples who are traveling a similar journey and emphasizes that maintaining self-esteem and self-worth are important for all.

William H. Kutteh, MD, PhD
Fertility Associates of Memphis

Introduction

I have learned everybody has a story but that many are not willing to tell it. This, I believe, is especially true when it comes to infertility. For many years I refused to let people enter my world of shame and embarrassment. It was not something I was proud to own, and I was not about to let people know of the challenge that I thought degraded me.

Not being able to have children can have a dramatic impact on one's life. I know because I suffered from infertility, which impacted me in ways I could never have imagined. It had a life-altering, gripping effect that changed the very way I viewed myself and those around me. The effects of infertility are not easily understood by those who have not experienced it.

During my infertility battle, my focus was primarily on what I felt had gone wrong or what I thought I could not have. I became so consumed with my emotions that I forgot about the many wonderful things that I had in my life. Because of its all-consuming impact, I missed out on many of the great gifts life had to offer me. My infertility became so overwhelming that the joys of life no longer mattered.

I wanted to create life with my husband and feel that life growing inside of me. I wanted to experience that mother-child bond I had heard so much about. I longed to know what it felt like to hold my newborn child for the very first time and feel its tiny body on my chest. I wanted to be fruitful and add to our family tree.

The desire to conceive was so strong that it shook me to my very core. I wanted what my mother and my sisters had. As time went on, I witnessed my nieces and even my stepdaughter bring life into the world. With the birth announcement of each new child, my desire continued to grow, and my heart ached continually for what I felt I would never experience. They were able to accomplish something that I was denied. It seemed completely unfair and even cruel until the day I finally woke up. I awakened from my self-inflicted nightmare and began to see life in a more beautiful and enlightening way. It is that enlightenment that I have chosen to share with you.

Infertility is like being trapped in a room with no windows: all I could see was what was before me, and this is how I got stuck. I was sabotaging my own happiness, until I was able to acknowledge that even though what I was going through was indeed real and painful, life wouldn't be over for me if I never conceived and birthed children. After accepting infertility as a part of my reality, I slowly began to stop grieving and started the journey of moving forward. As time passed, I realized that the room that had held me captive now had windows and doors.

Overcoming the Emotional Stigmas of Infertility: Barren but Not Ashamed is a memoir of my personal journey through infertility. I share the various disappointing events that led me to accept a mindset of defeat and embrace a myriad of negative emotions and stigmas that, for a period of time, took power over my life. On the outside I appeared happy, carefree, strong, and confident, but behind that mask I hid shame, pain, hurt, self-ridicule, and constant disappointment that wasn't evident to many people, including those closest to me.

"Barren" is a biblical term that is not commonly used today as it relates to infertility, but it described my situation perfectly. Yet my womb was not the only thing that was barren. My hopes and dreams of having children, which many of the women in my family saw come true, had become barren, as well. I constantly wore a "damaged goods" label that presented itself with each disappointing realization. Along with that label came discouragement, self-pity, isolation, anger, sadness, loneliness, hurt, embarrassment, and a laundry list of other tormenting thoughts and emotions.

I was taught to be thankful for everything that happens in my life, but how could I possibly give thanks for being infertile? I lost touch with the real me and began to lose sight of the things that made me special. I devalued myself and could not see how anything good could possibly come from my circumstances. I definitely was not thankful and did not consider this to be a blessing. For this reason, I struggled with the concept of thankfulness for my infertility for a long time.

I was able to overcome my infertility stigmas and reclaim the power that I had previously relinquished, which allowed me to heal within and ultimately remove the mask that had kept me afraid and reluctant to speak openly about my truth. I was not only able to move beyond the damaging effect of my circumstances, I was able to recognize good in it.

The desire to rise above my situation sent me on a journey of looking deep within, rediscovering who I was and why my experience with infertility was purposeful. The process was empowering, and through it I learned that my journey was not just about me; it was also to help others who are suffering. The concept of being grateful for all things had a greater meaning for me, and it all made sense. Instead of focusing on my pain and disappointments, I learned the importance of being thankful for every part of my life, including my infertility journey.

Perhaps there are similarities between my experiences and the ones you are encountering. I am sharing my story because there are many women and men who are struggling with the inability to have children and are embarrassed or ashamed by it, like I was. Others are dealing with the torments and emotional stigmas associated with it, just as I did.

In this book, you will learn the emotional coping mechanisms and strategies for infertility that I used to overcome negative emotions and stigmas. These techniques allowed me to break free from my own tormented thoughts and gave me the power to remove the mask that kept me hidden for many years. It is my desire that you embrace the words in this book and allow them to help you during this trying period in your life. It is also my hope that you find a purpose in your infertility challenges.

You may be wondering if this book is for you. If so, consider the following: If you have ever longed to have children and were told your chances were slim to none, this book is for you. If you feel an empty feeling in your heart and a void in your soul every time you see a pregnant woman or a family with children, this book is for you. If you ever feel like giving up on conceiving but need the strength to go on, this book is for you.

If you have ever gone through a cycle of fertility treatments only to see your empty womb on the ultrasound screen and felt the sting of disappoint, this book is for you. If you have ever conceived a child and lost it from a miscarriage, this book is for you. If you are a man and have been diagnosed with infertility, this book is for you. If you are a husband or a loved one who shares in the heartache of a person facing infertility, this book is for you. If you are a stepparent, this book is for you.

If you feel embarrassed because you have fertility challenges, this book is for you. If you have felt heartache after seeing another negative pregnancy test, this book is for you. If attending baby showers has become too difficult, this book is for you. If you have dealt with infertility on any level, this book is for you.

Infertility is one of the most common medical issues for women and can cause heart-wrenching feelings. Its reality can make a person feel incomplete and ashamed. African American women have been stereotyped as being highly fertile, but infertility is quite prominent in this community. I have learned that more and more people from this ethnic group are being diagnosed with infertility. *Women's Health* magazine states that infertility affects at least 12 percent of all women up to age forty-four. Studies suggest Black women may be almost twice as likely to experience infertility as White women. That being said, the belief that any ethnic group can easily conceive is being challenged, and the dream of starting a family doesn't happen as easily as one may think.

Infertility is commonly associated with women, but a large percentage of men are diagnosed, as well. According to the American Society for Reproductive Medicine, "New studies show that in approximately 40% of infertility couples, the male partner is either the sole cause or a contributing cause of infertility." It is my belief that infertility threatens men's virility and masculinity. I believe they can hide behind a mask that can be as emotionally impacting as a woman's, if not more so.

I decided to use my life story as a means to help others move forward in their journey. I am a certified professional coach, an energy leadership index master practitioner, a member of the International Coach Federation, and have more than twenty years of personal infertility experience. Becoming an infertility and life-purpose coach allows me to assist those who are facing the turmoil and difficulties of infertility. This gives me the opportunity to help them sort things out; get unstuck; and find balance, endurance, and acceptance during their journey. I also lead a monthly infertility support group in my area.

I understand that everyone's experience with infertility is extremely personal, so I will not say that I know exactly what others have encountered or are feeling. I only know what I have experienced and that my infertility challenges led me to evolve into a stronger and better person. Without them, I would not have the experience and compassion to help others in their journey.

Infertility is like a thief in the night. It can rob you of your life. I let it rob me of mine for a very long time, but I found the strength and courage to stop it from stealing another moment of my peace, joy, and happiness. I am now stronger, wiser, more courageous, and free. It is my hope that by learning from my experiences, you will let go of any unproductive emotions and reconnect with the strength, courage, peace, and power that dwells within you.

CHAPTER 1

Be Fruitful and Multiply

Then God blessed them and said,
"Be fruitful and multiply."
—GENESIS 1:28, NEW LIVING TRANSLATION

I was born the seventh daughter and the ninth of ten children. My mother conceived and birthed seven girls and three boys, all of which were single births. Three of my sisters, Bernice, Earnestine, and Betty Ann, died as infants prior to my birth. I would hear their names mentioned from time to time in brief conversations by my older sisters, and I gained the most insight about my deceased sisters from them.

My dad and mom, Jeffrey and Lucille Rowell, were married in January 1951. Daddy was a big talker, very charismatic and friendly to everyone he met. He was easygoing and had a big laugh. Compared to Daddy, Momma was a woman of few words, but she carried a great deal of strength and wisdom. She was feisty but had a warm and caring smile that would brighten up your day. Momma called Daddy Bud, and he called her Cille. They loved each other dearly and were very happy together.

A few months after their wedding, Momma conceived their first child, and they were very excited. But something went terribly wrong during the delivery, and Momma became very sick. Her blood pressure got extremely high. The doctor told my dad that he could save only one of their lives, Momma or the baby.

Daddy had to make a quick, very difficult, and no doubt, scary decision. He told the doctor to save Momma's life. With that decision, Momma lived, but the baby was born dead. They named her Bernice. My mom had carried a healthy child to full term, went into labor, went to the hospital to give birth, and in the end, lost the child. I cannot even fathom what she must have felt upon learning that her child had died. I am sure the decision my dad made that day weighed heavily on his mind for quite some time, but without it, neither I nor any of my brothers and sisters would be here today.

After losing her first child, Momma later conceived and delivered two sons, Stanley and Eugene, and a daughter whom they named Vergie. Things were going well for them, and they were building a strong and healthy family. With great excitement and anticipation, Momma conceived and birthed another girl, whom she and Daddy named Earnestine. Sadly, Earnestine died a few weeks after being born, and once again, a dark cloud hovered over the family.

Approximately two years later, their sixth child, a daughter they named Delois, was born. Not long afterward, child number seven, a daughter named Betty Ann, joined the family ranks. The only feature about Betty's appearance that my oldest sister, Vergie, remembers is Betty's thick, curly hair. Her two big brothers nicknamed her Penny after a character on a cartoon show they loved. I do not know the reason, but Betty became very sick and lived only three months.

Brenda, child number eight, was born, and I, number nine, came along approximately three years later. Finally, Jeffrey Jr., child number ten and the youngest of us all, arrived on the scene. Daddy was fifty-one and Momma was forty-one when I was born and was forty-four when my younger brother was born.

The Rowell family was considered complete. Although there were lots of ups and downs, joys and heartaches along the way, I believe that the loss of our parents' three daughters was the main reason that family was so important to them and why we were raised to be so close. I don't recall my parents ever speaking about Bernice, Earnestine, and Betty Ann. I assumed it was just too difficult for them to talk about.

After I grew older and learned of my deceased sisters' existence, I should have asked my parents about them, but I never inquired, even after I became an adult. Although they were my sisters, they didn't seem real to me, especially in my younger years. They were names of people I did not know and had never seen. I wish I had taken the time to learn more about them from my parents when I had the chance.

Even though I hadn't known them, I never forgot their names as the years passed. They were my big sisters, three people whom I wish had been in my life. I think of them at times, and wonder how they would have looked or what they would have become if they had lived. What type of advice would they had given me? How many jokes and secrets would we have shared? How can you miss someone you have never met? I's not as hard as one may think. We were and are attached by the love of two parents who gave us life. That kind of love never fades away.

CHAPTER 2

Family Values

Families are the compass that guides us.
They are the inspiration to reach great heights,
and our comfort when we occasionally falter.
—BRAD HENRY

Being the youngest of four surviving daughters was quite an experience. I received a great deal of love and attention, and my older brothers and sisters always looked out for me. They even made sure that no one—other than they—picked on me. I felt safe with them. There were rivalries and tauntings by my brothers (one in particular), but I suspect they were no different from those of any other family.

One of our parents' biggest values was respect. We were taught to have respect for them, for our elders, for one another, for ourselves, and for everybody else. We were taught patience and forgiveness and to treat others as we wanted to be treated. Another important value in our home was family. These core values impacted my life in a major way. I secretly vowed that one day, when I had children, I would instill the same values in them.

Our parents were sharecroppers in the Deep South of Mississippi. Needless to say, money was often scarce. We lived in an old wood-framed house on the property that they farmed. While we lived a humble lifestyle, and family, love, and God—not necessarily in that order—were our top priorities. My oldest brother was often quoted as saying, "Our family didn't have a lot of money, but we were rich in love." How right he was. The love that our parents demonstrated each day through their example is what made me want to become a parent.

Daddy and Momma sacrificed a lot for us. There were times when they would go without to make sure we had what we needed. I was told that sometimes they wouldn't eat in order to make sure there was enough food for us. As a child, I never knew we were poor. I was happy and had my family. That's all that mattered to me.

Being in a large, family-oriented home heavily influenced me. Birthdays, Easter, and Christmas were always celebrated. Christmas was always my favorite holiday, and it was a true representation of family closeness. Momma would spend days baking cakes and pies, making the house smell so wonderful that we could barely contain ourselves. I couldn't wait to taste them.

Dad would buy a variety of assorted candies, such as old-fashioned Christmas candy, peppermint candy canes, orange candy slices, and candy corn. He would also buy lots of apples, oranges, and Brazil nuts for him and the kids to snack on. Every year, these goodies were hidden in a special place within the confines of our home. We could never find his hiding place, but we could always smell the fruit.

Dad would go out into the woods and chop down a Christmas tree, which he and the older children would decorate. The younger children would each be given our own "Christmas box." They weren't anything fancy, just simple packing cardboard boxes that he got from the grocery store, but to us, they were special. We would write a note to Santa on the outside, telling him the special gift and the number of apples and oranges we wanted. When we awakened early on Christmas morning, we would find what we had requested inside the box. As an extra gift, we also got several sparklers. Our dad would light them one by one as we watched the sparkling show. I loved the way they looked. It made Christmas magical.

What holds most in my memory was the special prayer we did as a family. We all crowded together, kneeling in our tiny living room, which was also part of our parents' bedroom. Heads bowed and eyes closed, my dad would lead us in a very, very, very long prayer of thanksgiving. The prayer probably wasn't as long as it felt, but to a young child it seemed like an eternity.

Daddy took long pauses in between his prayer phrases, so I was never sure if the prayer was over or if he was searching for the next thing to say. I recall one Christmas in particular when I was about five years old. I wondered if that prayer was ever going to end. He took one of his elongated pauses, and I waited for what seemed like forever for him to say the next word, or some sign of his continuing. When no more words came forth, I looked at my two-year-old brother, smiled, and yelled, "Let's get up and play!" and immediately jumped up to run to my toys. Momma, who was kneeling next to me, quickly caught me and brought me back to the bedframe, where we had been kneeling. In my defense, I thought he was done, but I learned that day that prayers in our family ended in "amen," and until we heard that word, we stayed put.

I often think of that moment, sometimes smiling, sometimes laughing within. Even now, as I am writing, I can hardly contain the smile on my face. I feel such a glow. I can feel the warmth of the love and closeness in that tiny room. It is a memory I will forever hold dear to my heart. We didn't have a lot of things growing up, but we had love and each other. It was that closeness and the lessons our parents taught us that sparked the desire for me to one day have a large family of my own.

Questions to Ponder

1. What values from your family are most important to you?

2. Why are they important?

3. How have these values impacted your desire to have children?

CHAPTER 3

How It All Began

The beginning is the most important part of the work.
—PLATO

When I was in high school, I fantasized about the day I would marry the man of my dreams and have a family. My husband would be kind, loving, caring, charismatic, and gentle, just like my dad. He would also be fun, have a terrific sense of humor, and love to dance. I hoped he had a terrific voice and would sing romantic love songs to me.

Prior to my twentieth birthday, I decided to add an important qualification to my dream man: my husband would love children as much as I did. I wanted to have five, and I even began to pick out their names. We would have a great life and a fairy tale happily-ever-after ending. This seemed reasonable to me. My mom and dad had a great marriage and happy family, and so would we.

Three years after finishing high school, I went to a small two-year college in Mississippi and majored in accounting. I graduated as an honor student and then enrolled in a four-year institution in the same state. I hoped to have a serious relationship, and began to wonder when I would meet Mr. Right. I was twenty-four years old.

I lived in the college dormitory and made several good friends. Being somewhat reserved, I was not the type of person to talk about things with my friends or roommates that I felt were too personal. We mostly talked about our relationships, classes, and other college-related interests and events.

I didn't pay a lot of attention to my body or the intricacies of my monthly cycle. All that mattered is that it showed up on time. Since I didn't talk about it to anyone, not even my mom or sisters, I didn't know what was considered abnormal. My menstrual cycles were indeed heavy, but I thought that was normal and didn't give it much thought.

I finished undergraduate school and went on to enroll in the university's graduate accounting program. As a graduate student, I decided it was time to move out of the dormitory, so I shared a rented house with two college friends. While living there, I started having severe menstrual cramps. I didn't know the origin, but they were so painful at times that I could barely walk. I recall instances where I would literally have to crawl from one room to another. I was twenty-six or twenty-seven years old.

I only felt the severe cramps during the first day or two of my cycle, and then they would go away. I thought my body was changing and that this was part of the process. Since the pain ended after a couple of days, I didn't think it was serious enough to go to a doctor. This became my new normal, and life continued as usual. I came from a large family, so it never entered my mind that something was wrong with me and that having children would become an issue.

I was not in tune with my body and did not recognize that it was giving me signals that something was wrong. If I had not been oblivious to those indicators, perhaps the issues that were forming could have been detected early. I should have paid more attention to my body and taken the time to learn what was normal and abnormal.

By the time I was thirty-one years old I had earned a bachelor's and two master's degrees. I found a job as an accountant in Memphis, Tennessee, and after commuting for three months, I relocated to the city. In October 1997, I was introduced to a kind man named Chris Jones. We met through a friend at my job. Being new to the city, I was looking for someone whom I could trust to do minor repairs on my car. My friend assured me that Chris would do a great job and could be trusted.

I had not yet found a church, so I visited various ones in the city. On Sunday, October 26, I attended my friend's church. Although it was not a planned meeting, Chris and I showed up at the church on the same day. He was supposed to have visited on the prior Sunday, but he had the wrong address and had gone to a different church. I didn't know who he was, but when I saw him for the first time, he seemed familiar to me. I couldn't shake the feeling that I knew him from somewhere.

Even the clothes we wore were similar. Chris had on a three-piece green-and-beige houndstooth suit, and I wore a two-piece black-and-white houndstooth skirt suit. We were introduced after church services and made small talk while I waited for my friend. During that conversation, I tried to figure out where I had seen him before. He was a minister, and I sang in the gospel choir in college and at my church in Mississippi, and traveled to various functions. I thought maybe I had seen him at one of those events, but he had not attended any of the ones that I mentioned. It turned out that we had never met.

Chris told me about his little girl, Gabby. He spoke fondly of her, and I could tell that he loved her very much. He told me of his experience in working with vehicles and that he would be more than happy to inspect my car so he could determine how to fix it. After several minutes of talking, I felt comfortable enough to give him my phone number so we could set up a time for him to inspect my car.

After three phone calls, I knew Chris was interested in me. I, on the other hand, was not interested in him. He seemed nice enough, but I was only interested in getting my car repaired. He did a great job on my car. I paid him and thought that would be the end of it, but we stayed in contact. We talked often on the phone and began to hang out. He brought pizza on Friday nights, and we watched movies at my apartment. He was nice and easy to talk to, but I only wanted him to be a friend.

I immediately recognized that Chris was a protector. Many times, before leaving my apartment, he made sure that everything was secure. As soon as he was home, he called me just to make sure I was okay. We stayed on the phone talking and laughing until I finally fell asleep. Occasionally, on nights when he did not come to visit me, he called just to make sure my apartment was properly secured.

I began to notice there was something different about Chris. He had qualities that I had not found in any of the other guys I had met. He sincerely cared about people. He would give money to those less fortunate and car rides to people who were stranded. Even though I was afraid to admit it, I was being drawn to him with each visit and phone call. We were friends for six months and then dated for six months before he proposed. My world was changing, and everything was beautiful.

Chris was pretty close to my fantasy dream guy. We had a lot in common, and I found that we were similar in many ways. He was comical and fun, and his eyes were kind and gentle. He had many qualities similar to my dad's, but what stood out most for me was that he had a good and compassionate heart. He could meet a total stranger, and you would think they had known each other for years.

We were both affectionate, and just like me, he loved children. Chris had full custody of his daughter and was working hard to provide for her. As a single dad, he sacrificed to make sure she had the things she needed. It reminded me of my parents doing the same for me and my siblings.

I recall a particular conversation with his dad after our engagement announcement, which validated Chris's love for children. His dad said, "Frances, Chris loves kids. You know what I mean?" I answered, "Yes, sir, I know."

"I mean, he really, really, really loves kids," his dad went on. "Do you understand what I'm saying?"

"Yes, sir. I understand."

I told Chris about the conversation, and we laughed about it for quite some time. His dad's message was not a subtle one; I would have to be completely clueless to miss the meaning behind it. Little did I know that our short, simple conversation would come to haunt me for many years to come.

In November 1998, at the age of thirty-two, I became Chris's wife and an instant mother. I had no idea of the journey I was about to begin.

CHAPTER 4

The Family Waltz

The truth is, I've been lucky. But just like the waltz,
life has its own rhythm of rise and fall.
—LEN GOODMAN

My mom and dad had a very special relationship. They were married for over forty years and were great examples of how parents should be. My dad was a friendly and talkative man. He loved people and was well respected by those who knew him. Many considered him to be a minister, but I never heard him say that of himself. Although Daddy faced many trials in his life, he was a man of faith and loved God. He spoke with a calm and sometimes quiet voice but had a loud, cheerful laugh.

My dad was an affectionate and giving husband. He would perform small acts of kindness to show Momma the love he had for her. For example, whenever he went to the grocery story, he always brought her something back, even if it was nothing but a bag of grapes. He constantly did things to show his appreciation for Momma. Daddy treated everyone like he had known them for years. He had a gentle soul.

My mom was different. She was not a big talker but loved to have fun, and played various family games. Momma was more reserved in showing affection in front of the children. She demonstrated incredible strength and faith. Momma sang while doing chores around the house, and we could feel the power of her belief.

Toward the end of his life, Daddy had a stroke that took a toll on his health. Momma cared for him to the best of her ability. When the doctors gave up on Daddy, she never did. She loved him dearly and stood by his side until the day he passed from this Earth. After he died, a part of her died with him. Momma would often stare at Daddy's picture on the wall and long to be with him again. She missed him dearly and often spoke of it. Their hearts and souls were truly connected.

I learned a great deal about love, strength, respect, stability, and commitment in a marriage from my parents. I also learned the importance of family. I always felt that my family was happier because we had each other. Knowing that my parents loved me made a difference in my world. Theirs were the traits that I vowed to exhibit and demonstrate in my marriage and home.

I wanted my children to experience the amazing love, values, and nurturing that influenced my life. It would be the foundation that our lives would be built upon. I awaited the day that I would meet the man who would become my husband. I envisioned him to be just like my dad. I knew that day would come and looked forward to it with great expectation.

It was a beautiful, warm fall day in November 1998, and excitement was in the air. Chris's and my wedding day had finally come. Several members of my family arrived at my apartment to help me prepare for the big event. But instead of their helping me, I found myself helping my wedding party get ready. I was so busy that I didn't have time to be nervous. Fortunately, my wedding coordinator made sure things flowed smoothly.

Getting everyone ready took longer than anticipated. As we rushed to the church, my heart began to pound. "I can't be late for my own wedding. I have to make it there on time!" We parked at the church, and I rushed in with my gown in hand. The wedding was scheduled to start at four o'clock in the afternoon.

One of the church members ushered me to the dressing room to assist with my wedding gown, hair, and makeup. I felt like a pampered princess. The photographer was occupied with taking pre-wedding pictures and was asked to not take any photos of me yet. Instead, he took photos of the wedding party and others who were in attendance.

I wanted a simple, elegant, down-to-earth ceremony. Our wedding colors were black and off-white. Attendees consisted mostly of children aged six and under, because of my love for them and because of the purity of their hearts. Their inclusion would usher in an atmosphere of innocence, sincerity, and fun.

Gabby was my junior maid of honor. My niece, CeCe, was the bell ringer. Olivia, Chris's niece, and Kesha, my niece, were the flower girls. My sister Brenda was the maid of honor. Chris's dad was his best man. That was the extent of our wedding party.

The pastor officiating the service sent a message that it was time to start the ceremony. My heart suddenly jumped a beat. The event that would forever change my life was about to begin. As the wedding party lined up in the entranceway, I stood listening to the music playing. One by one the party entered the sanctuary and stood in their designated area.

The bell ringer shyly and hesitantly entered through the door, and everyone stood. This was it. All eyes were on me as I came into the room. My dad was not alive to give me away; he had died five years prior, so Jeff, my youngest brother, stood proxy for him.

Jeff waited for me with his hand held out. He caringly took mine and walked me down the aisle. Chris and I looked at each other with so much love. He was the one I had waited and hoped for. My dream had come true. The ceremony was short, heartfelt, and sweet. It was perfect.

The guests went to the reception area while the wedding party and family took additional photographs. When Chris and I finally made it there, the room was filled with the sound of music, the scent of delicious food, and laughter. Friends and family near and far had come to witness and help us celebrate our union. We were starting a new journey together. Not only was I a new wife, I was also a new mother. I couldn't have been happier.

Chris and I left the reception and went to our new place to gather our things so we could go on our honeymoon. Gabby was upset that she had to stay with her mom while we were gone. She was only five, and far too young to understand why she couldn't go on the trip with us. I remember her crying while Chris and I made efforts to comfort her. We explained that we would only be gone a short while and would see her very soon.

Chris and I gave up our separate apartments so we could move into a new one together as husband and wife. We wanted to start our new lives in a different home. A week and half after the wedding, he and I were preparing for Thanksgiving, our first family holiday. As a new bride and mother, I couldn't wait for that day to arrive.

Coming from a large family, I was used to seeing a lot of food during the holidays, and this holiday was no exception. Although it was only me, Chris, and Gabby, I cooked an enormous amount of food. The dining room table was overcrowded with all types of selections. Little Gabby sat at the table with huge eyes and a big smile.

We gave thanks for the many blessings the Lord had provided us, including blessing us to be a family. Everything was delicious—except for the green bean casserole that Chris had made. Although he is an amazing cook, I made him promise never to make that dish again. It is a family joke now. Over the years, he has improved the recipe and is allowed to cook it occasionally, with permission.

From the moment I met him, Chris has displayed a giving and loving heart. I noticed his willingness to sacrifice comfort for himself so that Gabby could have what she needed. Witnessing the loving relationship Chris had with his daughter attracted me to him more than anything he could have said or done. I knew that same love would keep us bonded as a family.

Life was going great. The three of us were getting along and enjoying being a close family. Suddenly, we faced our first family crisis. Two months after we were married, Chris was hurt on the job; he sustained a back injury and was unable to work. As newlyweds, we had to make adjustments, including operating with one income. My being financially responsible for the entire family was unexpected. It was challenging at times, but with the help of God and being practical, we were able to overcome.

Spending time with Gabby was a pure joy. She was an inquisitive, smart, and talented five-year-old. I could tell that she was going to have a beautiful singing voice. Over the years, we sang in church choirs together. I would give her singing tips to help improve her talent. One of the things that made Gabby special was her caring and tender heart. At a young age, she prayed for homeless people and gave money to people in need.

Gabby was an excellent student and breezed through her classes, making all A's. One of the things she struggled with was penmanship. Her handwriting was like chicken scratch. In order to help improve it, I would have her sit at the kitchen table and practice writing sentences. She would whine, complain, and get angry with me, but I felt writing was just as important as her other homework assignments.

My greatest enjoyment in parenting Gabby was teaching her what I considered the important things in life and seeing her apply them.

She was a rising star who could not be ignored. My heart overflowed with joy and pride to see her growing into a beautiful young woman spiritually, physically, and scholastically.

I truly disliked disciplining Gabby. Chris and I preferred talking with her before considering other discipline methods. It hurt me to see the sadness in her eyes when she believed she had disappointed us. Chris and I knew Gabby would make mistakes, just as we did. We were proud of her accomplishments and the progress she was making. The main things we expected from her were respect and following the rules we set. We also expected honesty. Gabby was my darling daughter. Her smile lit up my day.

She had such a sweet personality and was so loving and adorable. I would take photos of her playing dress-up in my outfits. My clothes swallowed her little body, but she would smile and pose like they had been custom made just for her. Every year, I took a first-day-of-school photograph of her smiling and holding her new backpack. I looked for any excuse to take a photo of her, even if she was getting ready to brush her teeth. I wanted to preserve as many moments of our time together as I possibly could.

My employer hosted an annual family day picnic for the employees, and Chris, Gabby, and I looked forward to attending each year. It was a big event with lots of food and fun activities. We had such a great time taking photos, playing games, getting painted faces, and going on hayrides. We were exhausted at the end of the day. This was a time when the company demonstrated the importance of family and friendships. I was always deeply appreciative of their willingness to do something special for those who attended.

One year, Gabby received the chance to come to work with me in the accounting department. I explained my job responsibilities and gave her small tasks to complete. She was eager to learn and happy to help. I proudly introduced her to my colleagues. Soon, many people at the office knew her. She made a great impression. Afterward, my teammates repeatedly told me how smart she was. I wasn't sure what Gabby wanted to accomplish in life, but I knew it was important for her to understand that she had the power to succeed regardless of her situation. She had access to many opportunities. She only needed to choose.

My greatest desire was to give Gabby the same type of solid family foundation and nurturing as I had received as a little girl from my parents. I wanted to do my part in helping her to become a strong, confident, and independent woman. I desired for Gabby to have a happy childhood and to always feel safe. I wanted my little princess to know she was loved and that her dad and I would do anything within our ability for her. I wanted Gabby to appreciate life's blessings and to not take them for granted.

I could not wait to add to our family and thought it would happen right away. Growing up, I was blessed to have siblings my age to play with, and wanted Gabby to have them also. After I was diagnosed with infertility, I wondered if I would be able to give her that experience. Although Gabby never said anything about it, I felt she wanted a brother or sister. She was a real trooper and never complained. She was content being the only child, but it bothered me tremendously.

Gabby and I had a lot of great moments with plenty of laughs together, but I will not lie; it was not all snow cones and pop tarts. It was sometimes tough being her second mom. There were plenty of occasions of heightened frustration for both of us. I became the blame, the fall guy, and the target for her anger, especially when she was punished by her dad. I started noticing it when she was around eight or nine years old. If Chris either corrected Gabby or wouldn't give her something she wanted, she would get upset with me.

One occasion in particular comes to mind. The three of us were hanging out in our small kitchen one morning. I don't recall the conversation, but Gabby asked her dad for something, and he told her no. I was not involved in the conversation and had nothing to do with his response. Suddenly, I felt the urge to turn around, and when I did, I saw a frown and two angry eyes staring at me.

While intently watching my daughter, I thought to myself, *Why are you looking at me like that? This is between you and your dad.* Apparently, Gabby didn't see it that way. I was in the room, and suddenly it was my fault. I did not know the true origin of her anger that day. The odd thing was, she wasn't upset with me prior to her conversation with Chris, and we had not encountered any strife, either. Things had seemed fine.

This was the first of many such occurrences in our household. I soon began to witness the impact that divorce can have on a child. Although Gabby loved me, her true desire was to see her mom and dad back together so they could become a family again. She knew that would never happen as long as I was married to Chris. I was the threat that stood in the way of her parents reconciling.

I didn't know how she felt until about a year later, when Gabby admitted to me that she wanted her dad and mom to get back together. I said, "But if that happened, I wouldn't have anyone." She looked at me with sincere eyes and gave me the name of a man I could be with. She had it all planned out. Without thinking, I immediately said, "I don't want him."

My response caught us both off guard, and we immediately started laughing. I then lovingly held her and said that I understood her desire for her parents to get back together, but it was just as important that they be happy, too. I said that her dad and I were happy, and her mom was happy with her life, also. My heart ached to see the sad look on our daughter's face. She loved all three of us and was caught in the midst of the family she currently had and the one she secretly longed to have.

Gabby was such a sweet young girl. She didn't ask to travel back and forth between parents. But life happens, and sometimes marriages don't work out. I knew she was too young to understand this and probably wouldn't for many years to come. Even though she was happy most of the time, I knew there was a part of her heart that was broken.

Perhaps in time, it would become easier for her to accept. As her second mom, all I could do was comfort her, pray, and be as sensitive to her feelings as I could. "Step forward and back, turn and spin." This had become a part of our life and what I called our family waltz. Like a waltz, we went back and forth, sometimes drifting apart only to come back together again.

Just as things began to settle down, I knew that at some point in time, major adjustments would arise again. I knew that based on our family's rhythm, the speed would continually change the pace, motion, and direction of our dance.

CHAPTER 5

New Bride, New Mom

Blood doesn't always make a parent;
being a parent comes from the heart.
—UNKNOWN

After our wedding, I was ready to start having children right away. Even though I was over the age of thirty and had been sexually active in the past, I had never gotten pregnant. I wasn't always careful, so I considered it to be pure luck. Now that I was married, it was a perfect time to add to our newly united family.

Marrying Chris allowed me to become an instant full-time mom. Prior to our wedding, Gabby hung out with me while Chris attended to the prayer line at church. She and I would spend hours laughing, playing tickle monster and hide-and-seek in my apartment. We had built a relationship that I felt was unbreakable. Since Chris had full custody of his daughter, she would live with us, allowing more time to bond. I thought the world of Gabby, and we were very close.

Because Gabby was an only child, I thought it would be great to give her a baby sister or brother to play with. I was excited and nervous about becoming a new mom so quickly, but because of my love for Gabby, I knew our relationship would bloom even more.

I was always able to bond with children; it just came easily to me. I taught the children's Sunday school class at church and loved their energy and laughter. My wedding party consisted primarily of children. In one of my wedding photographs, I am completely surrounded by children, mostly from my Sunday school class, blowing bubbles and smiling. Being around them made me feel complete. It was one of the great joys in my life.

Becoming a new wife and mom was wonderful, but it did require a big adjustment. I was accustomed to living alone and being accountable only for myself. Now I had to learn to balance my work schedule with my new family as well as share parenting with Gabby's birth mom. Gabby visited her birth mom every other weekend. She looked forward to spending time with her and enjoyed having the best of both worlds.

I soon discovered that being a stepmom was not going to be as easy as I had envisioned. At first things went smoothly, but as time passed, it became more challenging.

I let Gabby decide what she wanted to call me. I never impressed any title or gave any preference. She chose to call me Momma, and as long as she was happy with that choice, so was I. I treated her as though she were my birth child, although I tried my best to not give the appearance of trying to replace her biological mother. I nicknamed her Shawty and worked faithfully to do my part to give her a happy life. Later on, I often wondered if her decision to call me Momma was the best choice, as I think it caused many of the conflicts that arose in our lives.

Some may believe that unless you are the birth parent, you are not a real parent. I have heard people say, "That's not her real dad," or "She's not his real mom." I question what people with this mindset consider to be a real parent. In my experience, being a real parent is so much more than what transpires throughout the birthing process. What occurs after the child has come into your life and the decisions that are made in their best interest are what define a real mother or father. Yet people often refer to the term "stepparent" as though it means less responsibility in the love, care, and upbringing of the child.

I can only say that my role as Gabby's second mom was a full-time responsibility. It included helping with homework, comforting her when she was sad or afraid, taking care of her when she was sick, nurturing, protecting, teaching, guiding, building up her confidence, and instilling in her the values that were instilled in me by my parents. I accepted that role and any challenges that came along with it. Indeed, there were many.

In 1999, I was so excited to celebrate my first Mother's Day as a new wife and mom. Gabby, not quite six years old, was happy, as usual. We all got dressed and drove to church in great anticipation of the day's events. I was a member of the choir; in between selections and while the minister was speaking, I periodically smiled at my husband and daughter in the congregation.

At the conclusion of the church services, I began hugging various choir members and making small talk. Then it happened. One of the female choir members walked up to me with a big smile and arms opened wide. As this was my first Mother's Day, I expected well wishes from her similar to those made by others in the church, but her message was not what I expected nor was prepared to hear. While hugging me she uttered, "Happy Mother's Day, even though you are not a real mother."

As I moved from her, I stood in total disbelief. How could anyone say something so inconsiderate? Surely, this was not intended to be a statement of endearment. Being told I was not a real mom simply because I was not a biological parent was insensitive, thoughtless, and cruel. Her reason for saying this to me was unclear, and although her words were hurtful and disappointing, I did my best to not let it ruin my special day. My new family was celebrating me, and that was what really mattered.

The reality was that Gabby had two mothers: one through birth, and the other through marriage. We both loved her, and we both deserved to be loved. Either one of us would move heaven and earth to make sure she was protected.

I was obviously not her birth parent, but I also did not feel like a stepmother. I was her second mom, the person who would love, support, comfort, and help her in this world. I was not trying to replace her natural mom. I only wanted to find a special place in her life and be there when she needed me, and even when she felt I wasn't needed. I was her second mom during times of celebrations, happy moments, rejections, anger, resentment, and frustration.

That was the position I stood upon when she was a little girl, and it is where I still stand today. I loved Gabby even during times when I didn't feel loved, wanted, or appreciated by her. She was my daughter. I prayed for her continually, punished her when needed, rewarded, mentored, consoled, and uplifted her the best I knew how. I cried many times along the way but somehow always found the strength to endure. If that is not being a real mother, then I don't know what is.

A few months after our wedding, Chris and I had been trying to conceive with no success. I began to have concerns that something was wrong. Why hadn't I conceived yet? Maybe I was just being paranoid. Maybe I was too anxious. Perhaps I wasn't giving myself enough time. I finally had a long discussion with my husband and decided to find out if my concerns were valid.

It's amazing how certain statements can find their way back to a person at the most inconvenient times. From the crevices of my mind, the words spoken by that church member began to surface. "You are not a real mother." They began to echo over and over. *You are not a real mother. You are not a real mother. You are caring for this child, but you are not her real mom.* Thinking of my beautiful little girl, I could only respond, "Oh, yes I am."

CHAPTER 6

This Can't Be Real

It's going to be okay in the end.
If it's not okay, it's not the end.
–ANONYMOUS

At the age of thirty-one, I informed my gynecologist that I was having a lot of soreness in my lower abdominal area during the first couple of days of my cycle. In June 1998, she referred me to a physician to try to determine the origin of the pain. The physician examined me and said that my uterus was normal in size, although she did notice that I was in pain when she moved my cervix.

Her diagnosis was pelvic pain and possible low-grade pelvic inflammatory disease. She gave me two prescriptions, one of which was for clearing up the pelvic inflammation. I was to take the other as needed for the first forty-eight hours of my menstrual cycle. After three cycles, she instructed me to return to see if there were any changes in my symptoms.

Upon returning in October for a follow-up appointment, I informed the doctor that I was still having pelvic pain during the first few days of my menstrual cycle. My cycles were very heavy, and I experienced a considerable amount of discomfort. The doctor wanted to perform a pelvic ultrasound to rule out the possibility of fibroids or cysts. She also instructed me to take prenatal vitamins to help with iron-deficiency anemia.

A technician performed the pelvic ultrasound two weeks later. After the test was completed, she told me that she would fax the results to my doctor and that I would need to speak with her for additional information. My doctor told me that the ultrasound showed an enlarged right ovary. It measured 4.9 cm x 3.6 cm, and there was a 4.1 cm cyst. The doctor said that there was no need to take action on the cyst, but she would monitor it to see if it would shrink on its own.

During a routine breast examination in November of that same year, a lump was discovered in my left breast. My doctor schedules a bilateral film screen mammography and breast ultrasound. The ultrasound showed a two-centimeter mass that was consistent in appearance with a fibroadenoma, a noncancerous breast tumor that most often occurs in young women. Several other smaller masses were also noted. Two eight-millimeter cysts were discovered in my right breast and were thought to likely be the same. My doctor recommended a surgical consult for further evaluation.

Fibroadenomas are relatively common, but based on the consultation assessment, the doctor felt it would be a good idea to have the two-centimeter mass removed. I was not overly concerned with the lump mainly because I had had a similar procedure done in my early twenties. Still, it was a lot to deal with when combined with my pelvic pain problem.

Surgery was scheduled for December 1998, and the mass was removed from my left breast. The surgery was successful, and the lump was removed and confirmed as benign.

My next follow-up appointment was in early February 1999.

Chris and I had been married for two and a half months, and we were actively trying to conceive. I continued to take the prenatal vitamins each day but discontinued taking another prescribed medicine because it made me nauseated. I reported to the doctor that I still experienced pelvic pain.

Another follow-up pelvic ultrasound was scheduled for the last week in February 1999 to see if there were any changes to the right ovary cyst. Based on the ultrasound results, a 3.8 cm hemorrhagic cyst was detected. As I understand it, a hemorrhagic ovarian cyst is an abnormal growth formed as a result of bleeding into a follicular cyst. Because the ultrasounds were done four months apart, the doctor could not be sure if this was the same cyst or a newly formed one.

For the moment, we made no additional plans concerning the cyst. The doctor would just monitor it to see if any changes occurred. Other than that, life at home was good. I was enjoying being a new bride and mom. We all were bonding and learning more about each other with each passing day. Gabby was a few months shy of her sixth birthday and was carefree, happy, loveable, and cute as could be. Chris was charming and fun to be with. The time we spent together was magical. I had never been this happy, and felt that life could only get better.

March 4, 1999, started out as a normal day. Chris and I went to work, and Gabby went to kindergarten. It was not a stressful or demanding day. Nothing at work occurred out of the ordinary. When we came home, Chris and I made dinner together. After we had eaten dinner, I reviewed Gabby's homework.

Later that night, something changed. I began to have excruciating pain in my pelvic area. It was so intense that my husband rushed me to the emergency room. I was bent over in pain and crying fiercely. I was not sure what was going on, but it was the worst pain I had ever felt in my entire life. As the medical staff attended to me, I could tell that Chris was very worried. I lay on the gurney feeling helpless, and I was not prepared for what was about to occur.

I could not have imagined the pain getting worse, but when the emergency room medical staff began to do a pelvic exam, I screamed out in agony like I had never done before. I thought, *This can't be happening! What's going on? What's wrong with me?* I do not recall much after that. I do not know what triggered the pain that night, nor do I know what was done to alleviate it. I assume the emergency room physician gave me strong pain medication.

I hoped that I would never have to go through that type of suffering again. Thankfully, since that night, I haven't had a repeated experience of pain to that degree.

I found out later that because of the severe discomfort I was experiencing, the emergency room staff tested me for sexually transmitted diseases, which came back negative. My primary care physician received my emergency room test results, and hoping to get a better understanding of the origin of my problem, she referred me to a doctor at one of the medical groups in the city whom I will call Dr. John.

We had a discussion about the cyst that was found on my ovary. Four months had passed between the time the four-centimeter cyst was detected in October 1998 and the one discovered in February 1999. I told Dr. John that the cyst was large enough for me to see and feel under my skin. I also told him that I had been having persistent right-side pain most of that time.

I was thirty-two and had never been pregnant. I expressed my concerns to the doctor about not being able to conceive. I said that I had not used contraception since 1991 and had only been intermittently sexually active during that time. I told Dr. John that my husband and I married in November 1998 and had been trying to conceive, with no success. He and I talked about infertility during the session. He said that other than the pelvic pain and the ovary cyst, I was in good health.

Since I had been having pelvic pain for quite some time, Dr. John discussed the option of having a laparoscopy. He would use this diagnostic surgery to investigate the ovarian cyst as well as perform an evaluation for future fertility. He arranged a follow-up ultrasound to review the pelvic pain and right ovarian cyst formation. The ultrasound showed that the cyst on the right side was gone, but due to other irregularities he had discovered, as well as my fertility concerns, he scheduled a laparoscopy.

Dr. John performed the laparoscopy on April 12, 1999. The results from that procedure marked a turning point in my life that I was not prepared for. It confirmed the concerns that I had. There were indeed complications that interfered with my ability to have children. I was at a loss for words. *This can't be real,* I thought. But it was my new reality, one that I would face for many years to come.

CHAPTER 7

Starting Fertility Treatments

Let your hopes, not your hurts, shape your future.
—ROBERT H. SCHULLER

I was nervous about the laparoscopy procedure, but my husband and mother-in-law were there to provide me with comfort and support. After I woke up from the procedure, Dr. John came to the recovery room to tell my husband and me what he had discovered. The laparoscopy revealed a severe and extensive case of endometriosis. I thought, *Endometri-what? What did he say?* I remember him saying that it was so severe that both of my ovaries were literally glued to my back, and the only thing he could do was to try to unstick them. There was scarring and adhesions everywhere. The entire cul-de-sac was obliterated with two enlarged and swollen ovaries. The endometriosis affected both of my fallopian tubes, as well. Dr. John injected blue dye into both of my tubes. The right tube drained the dye, but the left tube did not.

Chris and I met with Dr. John on April 20 for a postoperative examination. We reviewed the photographs from the surgery as he talked about the findings from the laparoscopy. We discussed the

43

severity of the endometriosis in greater detail. I then understood the origin of the severe pain I had been experiencing dating back to when I was in college. The doctor's plan was to use six months of Lupron therapy to treat the endometriosis and then attempt a pregnancy.

He explained that the Lupron would mimic early menopause. He also told me about the side effects of using it. The goal was to kill the endometriosis by stopping the menstrual cycle, which is part of its life source. As part of our fertility evaluation, my husband would need to provide a semen analysis to confirm there were no issues resulting from his prostate surgery when he was nineteen years old.

Chris and I visited Dr. John's office on May 18 to discuss my experience with the Lupron injection as well as the result from Chris's analysis. I had experienced some unusual bleeding during my first month of Lupron and wanted to make sure everything was okay. The doctor reassured me that there was nothing to be concerned about. He said that Chris's semen analysis came back normal and reflected absolutely no issues. That was good news. We now had to work on getting my condition corrected. I was glad to have an explanation for what was happening in my body and a plan in place to resolve it. Hopefully, Chris and I could get on with our lives and start building our family like we wanted.

In November 1999, after six months of using Lupron, I visited Dr. John's office to find out if the treatment had worked. I told him about some of the side effects I experienced while using the drug. He then examined me and said afterward that I would try Clomid for a few months to see if I could get pregnant. Things were looking positive for the first time, and I was feeling hopeful and excited. As instructed, I started 50 mg of Clomid on day five of my cycle.

I returned to the doctor's office on December 10 for my first Clomid check. Sadly, my cycle had started that day, which confirmed the negative home pregnancy test I had taken. I was concerned about the bleeding I was experiencing and wondered if it was related to an actual menstrual cycle or if it was an implantation bleeding. The doctor said he would check my hormone levels to confirm, and the test reflected a non-pregnancy. Feeling disappointed, I started on round two of 50 mg Clomid on day five, December 14.

I didn't know what to expect from the fertility treatments, nor was I mentally prepared for the constant ups and downs that came along with it. I had no idea trying to get pregnant could be so complicated and invasive. My emotions were on a constant roller coaster. It seemed unfair that something that seemed so easy for most women was challenging for me. I sensed a twinge of resentment and envy whenever I saw a pregnant woman, which was out of character for me. I was always thrilled to hear pregnancy announcements, but now I wasn't feeling so jubilant. I felt frustrated. Immediately recognizing that I didn't like feeling this way, I tried my best to push the emotions aside.

I went to Dr. John's office on January 31, 2000, for another Clomid check. After completing my examination, the doctor ordered a pregnancy test. To my dismay, the test results came back negative. This time, I was instructed to restart Clomid on day five at 100 mg per day for five days. I anxiously waited to see what would happen. Maybe the increased dosage would yield better results.

There were many back-and-forth trips to the doctor during the Clomid treatments. I was so focused on the fertility process that I barely noticed the amount of time that had elapsed. In what seemed like a blink of an eye and the twirl of a hand, a year had passed with no success of my conceiving. The Clomid didn't work, and I was left to wonder where would I go from there. It had been almost two years since the laparoscopy procedure had unveiled the horrific endometriosis diagnosis. Thus far, nothing the doctor tried had worked.

With each negative pregnancy test, my heart sank more and more. As I watched my nieces and nephews grow up, I wondered if I would ever be able to add to my new family. Most days were better than others, but as much as I had hoped something would be different, each passing month remained the same. In addition to the constant disappointment of not getting pregnant, I continued to suffer with the pelvic pain the first few days of each month. I found that emotional pain and physical pain are not a great combination.

Being a private person, I kept many things hidden. I laughed heartily on the outside while hurting silently on the inside, so few people knew what I was truly feeling. On the brighter side of things, I had my sweet new daughter and wonderful husband to keep me occupied. Every time I looked at them, my faith that our family would grow was renewed. We were happy together. They brought joy into my life. They were the sunshine that brightened my sometimes dreary days.

I looked forward to the new year, and January 2001 arrived with the expectation of new possibilities and a fresh batch of optimism. After several unsuccessful pregnancy attempts, I was open to taking a different approach. I had befriended a woman at work who was also having infertility issues. During one of our conversations, she told me about another co-worker who had been visiting a fertility specialist in the city. If this person was willing to speak with me, I could learn more about the specialist. A few days later, I spoke with the individual, and she gave me the name of the fertility doctor.

That evening, I talked to my husband about the conversation, and we decided to make an appointment. The fertility specialist was named Dr. William Kutteh. He was well known and respected in his field. He was also accepting new patients. Hope began to re-ignite in my heart. Two years had passed, and I was now on the verge of being thirty-five years old. I wasn't really concerned about my age because my mom had me when she was forty-one and my brother when she was forty-four. In my mind, there was plenty of time.

As part of Dr. Kutteh's intake process, a fertility assessment needed to be completed. I shared that I had never been pregnant and had been trying to conceive for two years. I informed him that a laparoscopy procedure had been performed in 1999 that revealed endometriosis, pelvic pain, and other related issues. I disclosed that Lupron injections and Clomid were used as part of my previous fertility treatment plan. I also provided information on my husband's fertility history as well as the medical history of my family.

The next step was to have all of my medical records sent to Dr. Kutteh's office. A copy of my medical records was sent to Dr. Kutteh for review. Shortly afterward, I received a letter in the mail stating that my appointment with the doctor would be on February 9. Now I was really getting excited.

My first appointment lasted for an hour and half and consisted of a comprehensive history and examination. The initial diagnosis was endometriosis, cramps, and pelvic pain. Driving to work that day, I wondered what the future would hold for me and imagined various possibilities. Perhaps now there would be a way for me to conceive in spite of the fertility issues. Maybe . . . just maybe.

Since I was age thirty-five, I learned that a clomiphene citrate challenge test was going to be done as a means of assessing my ovarian reserve and to predict my future pregnancy success. I was instructed to call the fertility center on day one of my menstrual cycle and to take prenatal vitamins. On cycle day three, the nurse would draw blood for a serum "follicle stimulating hormone (FSH) and an estradiol test. An ultrasound would also be scheduled on day three.

I was prescribed ten tablets of Clomid 50 mg. Two tablets were to be taken daily from cycle day five through day nine. A blood test for FSH would be done on cycle day ten. I picked up the prescription on

February 25, 2001, and had an appointment on Monday, February 26. I started taking Clomid on February 28 and followed the protocol for the remaining days, as before. On March 5, cycle day ten, I went into the office for blood work.

My doctor decided that another laparoscopy should be performed. In order to prepare for the procedure, I submitted a short-term leave of absence to the company where I was employed. The doctor provided the purpose for the leave as well as other pertinent information needed for the approval process. The outpatient surgery was performed on March 1, 2001, at the East Memphis Surgery Center.

After the procedure, Dr. Kutteh informed my husband and me that the endometriosis was very severe; it was categorized as stage four with dysmenorrhea. I wasn't aware that there were various stages to endometriosis, or at least I didn't comprehend what they meant. An article from an online version of *Health* magazine (02/14/2019) states, "Stage four is the 'severe' stage of endometriosis. In addition to many deep endometriosis implants, there are large cysts on at least one ovary and many dense adhesions throughout the pelvic region." The culprit of my many years of pelvic pain still existed. I believed it was the major factor in my inability to conceive.

The first laparoscopic procedure done in 1999 revealed that both of my ovaries were literally glued to the back. This time, they were completely glued to the front. The doctor was able to unstick them, but not much else could be done. I was sent home the same day to rest and recuperate. A postoperative appointment was scheduled for March 8.

During the postoperative appointment, Dr. Kutteh explained in further detail about the laparoscopy findings. He showed Chris and me images that were taken during the surgery, four pages with four images per page. As I looked at them, I wondered if this attack on my reproductive organs would prevent me from ever conceiving. I didn't understand the full scope of the discussion, but I knew conceiving may not be as easy as I had hoped.

After the conversation, Dr. Kutteh gave me the photographs. I have kept them up to this very day. Even as I look at them now, I try to rationalize how the endometriosis occurred. I do not know how to explain what the images contained, but some looked as though they were large cysts. It looked pretty serious.

In mid-April, Dr. Kutteh began ordering tests to measure my FSH level and thyroid stimulating hormone (TSH) level to gain a better perspective of my situation, and devise a game plan for treatment. Very high levels of FSH can be a strong indicator of less successful pregnancy outcomes. The results from this test would be pivotal in my treatment plan. Later in the month, more lab tests were run. I still suffered with endometriosis pelvic pain. The doctor noted that the fertility treatment plan was FSH and intrauterine insemination (IUI). The process involved doing a double insemination. Per the doctor's instruction, I began taking prenatal vitamins and low-grade aspirin.

Dr. Kutteh wanted me to use Gonal-F (gonadotropin) 75 IU. He explained that by using this fertility medication, the risk of multiple pregnancy greater than twins was less than 3 percent. Chris and I were eager to have children and were not concerned with the risk factor. Before starting the therapy, my husband and I had to attend a gonadotropin injection teaching session. We also received a teaching video and injection kit to take home to review and study and become familiar with the process.

Chris and I were scheduled to meet with the nurse to demonstrate that we understood the proper mixing and injection technique. We were able to properly show our understanding of the technique and were cleared to use the medication. As part of the gonadotropin therapy, I was instructed to call the reproductive endocrinology nurse on my cycle day one if my period started before two o'clock in the afternoon. If it started after two o'clock, I had to call the next day. After speaking with the nurse, my first ultrasound and blood test would be scheduled on cycle day two or three.

My cycle started on Sunday, May 27, 2001. I was scheduled to come in on May 29 for an ultrasound and blood work. My treatment cycle is shown in table 1.

Table 1. Treatment Cycle

Cycle Day 1	Onset of menses. Start prenatal vitamins
Cycle Day 3	Ultrasound and estradiol blood test
Cycle Days 3,4,5,6,7	Inject gonadotropin 2 amps
Cycle Day 8	Ultrasound and estradiol
Cycle Day 8, 9	Inject gonadotropin 2 amps
Cycle Day 10	Ultrasound and estradiol blood test
Cycle Day ___	Day of hCG (Profas, Pregnyl usually induces ovulation within 12 to 36 hours)
Cycle Day ___	First IUI (approximately 12 hours after hCG)
Cycle Day ___	Second IUI (approximately 36 hours after hCG)
Cycle Day 32	Home pregnancy test (if no menses). Call office with results. If positive, come to office for blood work. Start vaginal progesterone 50 mg twice a day (two days after insemination)
Cycle Days 45–49	Sonogram will be scheduled to evaluate pregnancy.

I came in for my first ultrasound and estradiol blood test on cycle day three, May 29. The blood test was done to measure the concentration of estradiol in my blood. The ultrasound measured the number, size, and location of my ovary follicles. During this session, the nurse was able to take the necessary measurements, but because there was a cyst discovered on my left ovary, the cycle treatment had to be cancelled. I would have to wait a month before we could try again.

My next cycle day three was on July 6. As with the previous appointment, I came into the office for an ultrasound and blood test. The reproductive endocrinology nurse on staff measured my follicles and instructed me to start using two amps of gonadotropin. We mixed the medicine like we had been taught, and it was time to administer it. Chris made the first injection in my lower back area, at the top of my buttock. That was a scary experience for both of us, and it was different from practicing. This was the real deal.

During this treatment cycle, I also started taking the injections in my stomach area. I was so afraid that I would do it wrong, and needed my husband in the room for moral support, encouragement, and confirmation that I was doing it correctly. Chris made jokes to ease the uncomfortable feeling that I was experiencing, but I knew he was just as nervous as I was. He wasn't very comfortable giving me the injections, but we both knew that if we wanted to have a chance at having children, it had to be done. We were a team, and together, we could handle anything.

I continued using two amps of the injections per the daily instructions that I had been given. On cycle day eight, July 11, I returned to the office for another ultrasound and estradiol blood test. Things appeared to be going well. We continued with the two amp injection treatments and returned to the office on cycle days ten and thirteen for additional ultrasounds.

After my egg follicles became mature, I was instructed to take the hCG (Pregnyl) which was given to induce ovulation. Chris and I were scheduled to come in for our first IUI. Things were now moving in a positive direction. I was nervous but full of hope at the possibility of the treatment working. The IUIs were done on cycle days fourteen and fifteen, July 17 and 18. We had to wait to see if an implantation took place. This was thrilling and scary. I was extremely excited but nervous.

I envisioned the two of us announcing to our families that I was pregnant. I even put pillows under my blouse to see how I would look. I fantasized about someone throwing me a baby shower and receiving all of the wonderful congratulations and well wishes. I woke up each day with great anticipation and optimism. I went to work with a different attitude.

The two-week waiting period seemed to last an eternity, but it finally came to an end. When the test results showed that I hadn't conceived, that great anticipation I felt suddenly turned into a cold slap in the face. I was overtaken with utter disappointment. I had built my hopes up so high.

It never occurred to me that this treatment wouldn't work. Maybe Chris and I didn't mix the medication correctly. Perhaps we made a mistake when injecting them into my body. My mind searched for answers, a reason why it hadn't worked. The answer was that it was simply a failed attempt. This particular IUI cycle just didn't work, and I had to accept it. Dr. Kutteh decided to increase the gonadotropin to three amps during my next treatment cycle. It was time to start the process all over again.

Over the next few months, my husband and I went through a total of three cycles of IUI treatments. Although the dosage of medicine was increased in the hope of yielding better results, each treatment proved to be unsuccessful. Each time I lay on the examination table watching the nurse perform the ultrasound, I was reminded that my womb was empty. This caused a huge void in my heart. After the completion of each treatment, I felt the pain of seeing another negative pregnancy test result. Sometimes I hoped that the clinician was mistaken and that somehow, some way, I had conceived, but deep in my heart, I knew it was only wishful thinking.

No one in my family knew Chris and I were taking IUI treatments. I am not sure why I didn't tell them. Maybe I felt I would be criticized. Maybe I felt they wouldn't understand. After all, my three sisters were able to conceive without any assistance. It made me feel like an outsider, and in my mind only, unaccepted. It is amazing how certain situations can make us think that things that are completely untrue are real. I was able to go to college, earn several degrees, and make a good living, but the one thing that mattered the most continually escaped my grasp. My sisters were able to conceive, but I could not. I was envious of them and ashamed that I felt this way.

After the third failed IUI attempt, Chris and I decided to take a break from the treatments. It had become too much for me to handle. During that year, we wanted to take it easy and see if we could conceive on our own. Being at work was sometimes challenging as I listened to other women announce their pregnancies. I was sincerely happy for them, but it was often difficult to participate in their joyful chatter and watch the progression of their pregnancy. One colleague in particular kept and shared a photo album capturing how her body changed each month with the growth of her unborn child. She had no idea that each time she showed me the photos my heart would ache more and more. It was during this time that I first began to wear a mask to conceal my feelings.

The mask I wore reflected a countenance of happiness, but my true emotions were kept hidden behind it. My co-worker hadn't done anything wrong. She was only sharing her joy with the women she had befriended. How could she have known that her happiness was causing me sadness? My feelings remained a secret, and each month I rejoiced with her outwardly as I prayed inwardly that one day, it would be my turn.

Changes occurred at work that gave me the opportunity to clear my head and get away from the constant frustrations of failed pregnancy attempts. In 2002, my manager offered me a secondment assignment to work as a senior business analyst in New Jersey. This opportunity allowed me to travel quite a bit. I began the assignment by working two weeks in state and two weeks out of state for a couple of months. I was then asked to relocate to New Jersey for the duration of the project.

The company provided a furnished apartment, where I lived until the completion of the assignment. Being separated from my family was difficult and lonely at times. But because I was extremely busy, there wasn't a lot of time to focus on infertility and all of the disappointments that accompanied it. I was relieved but knew that I would eventually have to face my reality again.

I missed my husband and daughter very much. We talked every night before I went to sleep. Being separated from them was tough. I wasn't accustomed to being away from them for long periods of time. As a way to help deal with our separation, the company flew Chris and Gabby out to visit me for a week-long vacation.

It was so wonderful to be with them. We cherished every moment and enjoyed touring New York and Philadelphia. We had a lot of fun and thoroughly enjoyed the change of scenery. At the end of our vacation, they returned to Memphis and I continued focusing on the work I was doing.

Chris and I decided it was time to purchase our first home. We had been renting a house from one of his relatives for a year but wanted to have something of our own. The house that caught our eye was a three-bedroom, two-story home with a fenced-in backyard. We had bought a cute little Maltese named Angel, who made a great addition to our family. There was plenty of space for fun activities and a safe place for Angel and Gabby to play. Things were falling into place.

Since I was temporarily living in New Jersey when we were purchasing our home, I gave Chris temporary power of attorney to sign the contracts in my absence. With excitement, we closed on the house in May 2002. It was our first house, and we were very happy. Chris and Gabby had already been living in the house for a few days when I came home for a weekend visit. It was all so surreal for me.

We celebrated and gave thanks the entire weekend, and then I hopped back on a plane to New Jersey to finish up my assignment. Afterward, I rejoined my family and enjoyed our new home. I absolutely loved the house. It was spacious and only three years old. The neighbors were very friendly, and Gabby had already started making friends with the children across the street.

After being in our new home for a few months, I still had not conceived. Chris and I began to talk about whether we wanted to continue fertility treatments. I was no longer traveling, which allowed life to settle back to normal. We came into agreement and decided to continue treatments with Dr. Kutteh and his staff. I would call them after the Christmas holidays.

We returned in January 2003 to discuss additional fertility options. It had been a year since our last visit. I informed the doctor that a twenty-five-thousand-dollar lifetime maximum for fertility was now available through the employee insurance plan at my job. I also told him that I had left-over medicines from our last IUI treatment.

The three of us discussed and revisited the findings from my March 2001 laparoscopy. Dr. Kutteh told us that I had an elevated day three FSH of 9.3 and day ten FSH of 20. He explained that this could mean a decreased pregnancy rate and an increased miscarriage rate. He also informed me that my egg quality and reserves were low and that my odds of conceiving were not very good. He said that there were some things we could try, but they may not be successful.

As I heard those words, my smile began to disappear. I thought, *This doesn't make sense. My mom had me when she was forty-one and my youngest brother at age forty-four. This must be a mistake.* But it wasn't a mistake. Dr. Kutteh explained the IUI cycles and discussed with us the diminished success of attempting in vitro fertilization. The options presented to us were to either continue the FSH IUI treatments, start invitro fertilization (IVF), use donor eggs, or consider adoption.

Dr. Kutteh thought that the use of donor eggs would give us our best chance of success. He gave us a pamphlet on assisted reproductive technologies to review for consideration. Chris told him that we would go home to discuss the options and call back with our decision. After careful review of the pamphlet, Chris and I decided against donor eggs. If we were to have a child, we wanted it to be born with both of our genes. We also didn't want to get anyone else involved in the conception of our child. Chris and I didn't want to take the chance of anyone interfering in our child's life or with our family. Medically speaking, this may have been the best option for conception, but it just didn't feel like it was the right decision for us.

I contacted Dr. Kutteh's office to inform him that my husband and I would continue with the FSH IUI treatments, and if that did not work, we would try IVF. Although we were familiar with the treatment cycle process, it presented the same emotional ups and downs as it had previously. Eventually, because the IUI treatments were not fruitful, we felt it was time to pursue the IVF option. Even though Dr. Kutteh had informed me that my egg quality was not very good, my husband and I were still hopeful that we could conceive through IVF. That hopefulness proved to be short lived.

I soon discovered that Chris and I would not be able to obtain the funds for the IVF treatments. I was devastated. My insurance plan representative explained to me the deductible and out-of-network costs for the fertility treatments. She said that my husband and I would have to pay up front for the treatments as well as the necessary medicines. She said that the entire amount of twenty-five thousand dollars would have to be filed in order to get the deductible, then Chris and I would have to file an insurance claim to receive reimbursement of the funds. The news came as a shock to us. We would have to pay a very large amount of money in advance if we wanted to use IVF.

Chris and I no longer had the money to cover the IVF treatments. We had used our funds to purchase our home in the year prior. I thought if I could explain our situation to Dr. Kutteh, perhaps he could make a special exception on our behalf. I felt it was at least worth trying, and decided to contact his office.

Upon contacting Dr. Kutteh's office, I was told by his staff that unfortunately, the office could not make an exception for us. Receiving the news, I slowly hung up the phone and sat alone in silence. It felt like my world was crumbling around me. What would we do now? I was at a loss for words. Suddenly, without warning, the tears began to flow.

CHAPTER 8

Time to Say Goodbye

God grant me the serenity to accept the things
I cannot change, courage to change the things I can,
and wisdom to know the difference.
—REINHOLD NEIBUHR

After I finally composed myself, I contacted Chris and told him that Dr. Kutteh's office could not make an exception on our behalf. Knowing how heartbroken I was, he reassured me that everything would be okay. I knew in my heart that he was right, but my head hadn't yet received the memo. I still was trying to figure out if there was something that could be done. Maybe there was a way that we could come up with the money.

I knew going to my family wasn't an option. They didn't have the additional funds, and most of them didn't even know Chris and I were going to a fertility specialist. We had already used our entire savings as well as money from our 401K plan to purchase our first home. Applying for a loan wasn't feasible, either. I just couldn't figure out a way that would allow us to use the IVF treatments.

I needed time to clear my head and sort things out. After doing a lot of soul searching and praying, I finally accepted that this was a situation I could not change. I went to Chris and said maybe it was time to end the fertility treatments. He agreed that it was probably the right thing to do. As much as he wanted to have another child, I knew that he had agreed to the treatments mainly because he knew it would make me happy. I wanted to try it, and he was willing to do it for me.

Chris is such a loving and supportive man. He has always been in my corner, encouraging and helping me. While I went through the fertility treatments, I was never bitter, annoyed, or resentful toward him. There were times I knew he didn't fully understand what I was feeling or going through. I also knew there were risks involved with the fertility treatments, but I wanted a child so much that I was more than willing to take ownership of the physical and emotional responsibility that went along with it.

Every pain and discomfort, from medicine and surgeries, were in my mind, a small sacrifice in comparison to the reward I would receive if the treatments worked. I gave no thought or real concern about any potential side effects until I started experiencing the side effects of the Lupron injections, which were administered to kill the endometriosis that had overtaken my reproductive system. One of the biggest side effects I experienced using Lupron was that walking up and down stairs became difficult and painful for me. Was it worth the effort? In the beginning I thought it was, but afterward, I wasn't so sure.

Since I would no longer be continuing the fertility treatments, I needed to figure out what to do with the remaining Gonal-F medicine. I still had several amps stored in my refrigerator at home that I would no longer be using. Dr. Kutteh's office had informed us that it would last longer if kept there. I needed to find a way to move forward, have peace, and let go. With that in mind, I sat at my computer and wrote the following letter:

Dr. Kutteh,

Thank you for taking time out of your busy schedule last month to speak personally with me in great lengths regarding the type of services that would be provided to me at your clinic. Our discussion helped me to gain a better understanding of my special situation. You provided a suggestion to me that allowed me to become hopeful that I would receive the assistance needed to conceive.

I was informed by your staff on 3/6/03 that several portions of your services require payment to be paid up front, for which I would receive reimbursement by filing a claim to my insurance company. Unfortunately, I am not able to pay for the services up front. My husband and I recently purchased our first home and no longer have the funds required. I was under the impression that charges would be filed with my insurance company, which has allotted a $25,000 lifetime maximum for infertility.

Yesterday I asked Karen L. to speak with you and your staff to see if an exception could be made and was told that no exceptions could be made. I have to admit that I am very saddened to know that I will not be able to use your services.

In order to find some closure, I would like to donate the remaining medications that I had while trying to conceive through IUI. I have 16 amps of Gonal-F 75 IU. The expiration date is April 2003, but I have kept them refrigerated as you suggested. I am hoping that one of your patients who is not able to purchase their own medicine will be able to use them. I will find comfort knowing that I perhaps played a small part in helping someone else.

Once again, thank you for the services you provided to me during my attempts to conceive. I wish you much success in your new practice.

On the following Monday, I gathered up the remaining fertility treatment medication and drove to Dr. Kutteh's office. I presented the sixteen amps of gonadotropin and my letter to the office staff. I explained that I would no longer be able to continue receiving treatment. I stated my desire to donate my remaining medicine to someone who had a better chance of conceiving but couldn't afford the fertility drugs.

It didn't make sense for me to continue with the treatments. What was the point in my continuing, even with the IUI? They hadn't worked up to this point. I knew the reality of my condition. The overall chance of my having children, based on my fertility diagnosis, was not good. The likelihood of my conceiving was low, and even if I did conceive, the probability of having a miscarriage was high.

As I spoke to the office staff, tears began to well up in my eyes. I was overcome with emotions and could not hide my feelings from the person at the counter any longer. All I wanted to do was get away. Saying goodbye, I left the clinic as quickly as possible. I wanted to be brave and empowered, but I didn't feel that way. I felt broken, abandoned, and alone.

I couldn't help but wonder why the treatments didn't work for me. As I drove to work, the events of the prior years began to replay in my mind. It had all started with my having horrible, unexplained pelvic pain the first few days of my menstrual cycle each month. I had endured multiple surgeries and various fertility treatments in the pursuit of having a child. In the process, I suffered through joint pain, weight gain, mood swings, early menopausal symptoms, frustration, tears, up-and-down emotions, and repeated disappointments. When it was all over, I found myself at the same place where I started. The only difference was that I now knew the reason for the pelvic pain—which still existed.

Dr. Kutteh and his staff were wonderful. I truly appreciated everything they did to help us. It was time for me to let go and move on. I had to accept the things I could not change and realize that this part of my journey was complete. It was time to say goodbye and to be open to what the future held for me and my family.

A week after donating the fertility medicine, I received a letter from Dr. Kutteh's office thanking me for my donation. The letter stated that my generous donation would allow them to provide treatment to another couple in their effort to achieve a pregnancy. With my generosity, their goal may become a reality. Dr. Kutteh's letter made me smile. A sense of happiness suddenly came over me. For the time being, I had the strength to move on. I was making a difference in the life of another person. I felt hopeful to play a small part in making someone else's dream a reality.

CHAPTER 9

The Fertility Fairy

You may not control all the events that happen to you,
but you can decide not to be reduced by them.

—MAYA ANGELOU

Flying as fast as her little wings could flutter, she holds her sparkling wand tightly in her hand. Zooming here and stopping there, she leaves the gift of life for women near and far. Similar to Old Saint Nick, the Fertility Fairy touches lives in a special way. She doesn't leave gifts for children under the Christmas tree. Instead, she touches the womb of a woman, allowing her to bring a child into the world.

"Guess what? I'm pregnant!" I had heard those words from friends, neighbors, family members, and co-workers on many occasions for several years. It seemed as if everyone was having a baby—everyone, of course, except me. Fertility was not a stranger to the women in my family. My maternal grandmother had seven children. Her oldest daughter, my mother, birthed ten children. Momma's sisters were also blessed to be quite fertile. Two of them had several children. One birthed ten times. Another had seven children. Their half-sister had four children. I have three sisters, and all of them have children. I even have four nieces who have children.

As you can tell, the Fertility Fairy was a frequent visitor to my female relatives. Floating from house to house, she made possible the good news that conception had occurred. She worked tirelessly to touch the women whom I fondly knew. As I heard of each pregnancy announcement, I waited with great anticipation for her to visit my home.

The land of children was plentiful, yet my garden continued to remain barren. That was a tough pill to swallow. For many years, I have watched the women in my family, including my daughter, bring forth life into this world. As this occurred, I sat faithfully on the sidelines, watching, waiting, and wondering if it would ever be my turn. Every time I learned of a new pregnancy, my heart would sink a little more. I just could not understand why the Fertility Fairy hadn't graced my home with her presence.

How the Fertility Fairy chose those who would conceive was a mystery to me. It didn't seem as though her selection was based on any special criteria, such as race, nationality, social or financial status, or background. Personality was not a factor, nor was height, weight, beauty, or charm. There was no common denominator that caused anyone to stand out. It just didn't make sense.

I wanted—no, I needed—to find out why the Fertility Fairy chose one person over another. I had no idea how I would discover the criteria of her selection process. If I had the chance to meet her, what would I say? Would she grant me a special favor allowing me to conceive? That would be wonderful, indeed.

One night as I was lying in bed, I heard a strange noise outside. Curious to see what was causing the sound, I peeked out of my bedroom window. To my utter amazement, I caught a quick glimpse of what appeared to be sparkling wings fluttering by. Intrigued at the sight, I saw a figure land on the home to the left of our house. She zipped down the chimney with dazzling sparkles trailing behind.

As quickly as she had gone down the chimney, she flew back up and out. Smiling, and with an expression of satisfaction, she flew speedily by my home. Landing on the house to my right, she repeated the same process. Who was this, and what was she doing?

Hovering over my neighbor's house, she looked around, surveying the other homes nearby. It looked as if she were checking to see if anyone else should be visited. The fairy was just about to leave but instead stopped in mid-air.

I must have made a sound that caught her attention. Suddenly turning in my direction, she flew to my window. I held my breath, thinking she was about to come into my home. Instead she looked at me with a sad expression. As I stood there watching in awe, she quickly flew away.

It appeared as though she intentionally skipped over my house in her hurry to visit other women in the area. I wondered why my house was overlooked. Why didn't this fairy come into my home?

I awoke the next morning feeling puzzled. Had I been dreaming? Did I witness a phenomenon? This couldn't be real. I brushed it off and didn't give it another thought.

After some time had passed, I learned that my neighbor who lived in the house to the left of mine was having a baby. A year or two later, I learned that the neighbor who lived to the right was having her first child. Out of three consecutive houses, with mine in the middle, I was the only one who had not conceived. It felt like a cruel joke.

I suddenly recalled the night I saw the fairy. Could that have been the Fertility Fairy? I had written it off as a dream, but perhaps it wasn't. She came to my window but didn't enter my house. Why did she look at me with such sadness? I eventually discovered why the

Fertility Fairy could not visit me.

Many years prior, during my college years, I had received a visit from the Fertility Fairy's evil nemesis, the Infertility Nymph. Instead of bringing joy and happiness, the Nymph brings pain, discouragement, division, anger, low self-esteem, and drama to all she touches. Laughing heartily, she wreaks havoc in the lives of her unsuspecting victims. The Infertility Nymph feels no remorse nor carries any regret for her actions. Her only desire is to cause jealousy, frustration, and heartache by taking away the one thing many women yearn for, the chance to have a baby. I also learned that many other women had been robbed of the gift of childbearing by this cruel and unkind being. The Infertility Nymph causes some women to suffer in silence and others to feel shame and embarrassment. Many, including me, have fallen prey to her tactics.

In this fictional tale, I use the concept of the Fertility Fairy as a way of expressing how easy it seems to be for others to conceive. Similar to how pixie dust is used to help Peter Pan to fly, conception for many, especially my family, seemed almost magical. In reality, magic was not part of the equation.

The tale of the Infertility Nymph depicts the emotions that everyday women who are challenged with the inability to conceive experience in their daily lives. Infertility is very difficult. Some women who have never had problems conceiving may take their fertility for granted, yet the struggle of being fertility-challenged is real. A key component to understanding the plight of those who cannot have children include awareness, compassion, and sensitivity to their battle.

The emotional baggage that is associated with infertility must be discarded so healing can take place. There is no easy fix, and adoption is not the solution in all cases. As a matter of fact, the recommendation of adoption can be considered quite insensitive by some. Being intuitive to another's quandary can make a world of difference.

The truth of the matter is that some people have difficulty conceiving, while some, like me, are not able to conceive at all. I wish I could explain why this happened to me, but I am not certain. It is hard to know that others can have what you dream of having. But I learned that I could do one of two things: I can accept this as part of my journey and see what I can learn from it, or I can live a life of defeat. I eventually chose to learn from it.

Today, when I see women who are pregnant, I no longer carry frustration and resentment. I am back to being that carefree and happy person who rejoices and celebrates the livelihood and the wonderful miracle that these amazingly blessed women have received. The Fertility Fairy and the Infertility Nymph no longer have a negative effect on my life, emotions, or attitude. Because I was able to break free from the controlling effects of infertility, I am happy, fulfilled, and joyful. But this did not happen overnight.

CHAPTER 10

Accuserlina

You've been criticizing yourself for years
and it hasn't worked. Try approving of
yourself and see what happens.
—LOUISE HAY

I had an enemy for many years. She was cold, heartless, manipulative, and persuasive. Her words were so powerful that they caused me to change how I thought about myself. She often lurked in the corridors of my mind while playing havoc with my emotions. I came to know her as Accuserlina.

Accuserlina would raise her ugly head during times when things were not going well in my life. She had an awful habit of reminding me of my mistakes and holding them over my head. Accuserlina was a tormentor throughout my life. She was more than willing to tell me how I didn't measure up or couldn't accomplish a particular goal. She even went as far as to say that I would never conceive a child, and proudly provided me the reasons why I didn't deserve to get pregnant. She was a liar in her own right, but I was so consumed with her accusations that I could not recognize it.

I don't remember the day when Accuserlina first showed up, but most likely she was always there. Doubt, blame, guilt, and hopelessness were the results of her handiwork. She tried to convince me that I wasn't worthy to have children because I had broken promises to God and disappointed the most important people in my life. She also made me feel like I was the oddball sister because I was the only one who couldn't have children.

There were countless occasions when Accuserlina would proclaim that I wasn't a faithful daughter. Many years after my dad's death, I was tormented by the painful memory of Father's Day 1993. While in college, I joined a small local church in the city. I was excited to be in the services and was dedicated to the pastor, his wife, and their ministry. Instead of driving home from college on Father's Day that year, I decided to stay in the city and help out at church. I had planned to go home the following weekend to spend time with my dad.

That weekend never happened. My dad passed away the Thursday after Father's Day. I was devastated and completely caught off guard. Overwhelmed with grief and guilt, I made the drive to my parents' house. The guilt was too much to bear. I even dreamed that I was weeping furiously as I followed my dad, lying on a hospital stretcher.

I couldn't believe God would do this to me. I didn't go home that weekend because I believed I was needed in church and was doing something special for the Lord. I became very angry with God and began to rebel. I felt He had betrayed me. I knew in my heart that God was not at fault, but I was so hurt that I didn't know any other way to handle my pain.

I also knew that rebelling wasn't the answer but when you are overwhelmed with grief, better judgment can get thrown aside. I was eventually able to move past the anger, and although I asked God to forgive me, I didn't know how to forgive myself. I wasn't even sure I deserved to be forgiven. I carried that hurt and heavy weight within for many years.

As time passed, I found myself measuring the level of commitment and efforts I had made toward my parents. I was there to help them, especially whenever I was needed, but no matter how much I did, I never felt it was enough. I was fortunate to work for companies that gave me flexibility to take care of family matters when necessary, so I was the one who most often stayed long hours and spent nights at the hospital with our mom.

Whenever I came home to see my parents, my dad always asked me to sing to him. I didn't know the words to most of the songs he requested, but I would try to sing them anyway. I would also do funny things just to make them both laugh. These were precious moments that made our time together special. The visits home became less frequent after I married and became a full-time mom. I was absorbed in trying to adjust to my new life, but whenever I was needed, I was always right there without hesitation.

After my dad passed away, I would visit Momma as often as I could. She also came to my home for long visits. I looked forward to having her stay with me, Chris, Gabby, and our grandchildren. We would spoil her and give her the royal treatment whenever she came. It was always a joy to have her in our home.

My mom lived many years before she passed away, and her passing was another sad moment in my family's life. I recall the events that led up to her death. My mom was residing in Mississippi with Vergie, my oldest sister, for quite some time. On this particular evening, Momma had just finished eating ice cream with Vergie and Eugene, one of my brothers, when she went to retrieve her Bible from her bedroom so she could do some reading.

As she was coming back down the hallway, Vergie noticed that Momma was walking strangely while trying to hold herself up with the wall. Vergie realized that Momma had just suffered a stroke. She notified the rest of the siblings that she was taking Momma to the hospital in Memphis. I was babysitting my two oldest grandchildren, ages four and one, when I received the call. Gabby was working and needed me to keep them for her.

I told one of my sisters to let me know when they had arrived at the hospital and that I would get there as soon as I could. I didn't want to bring the small children to the hospital at night, and I wanted to wait until Gabby got off work. My three sisters were at the hospital in the small room with our mom. She noticed I was not there and asked for me. My sisters told her that I would be there as soon as I could.

Later that night, I received a phone call saying that Momma had slipped into a coma. I sent Gabby a text message explaining what had happened, packed up the children, and immediately went to the hospital. By the time I got there, Momma had been moved to ICU. I sat in the hallway outside of the ICU and waited to see her. When Gabby left work, she came to the hospital to pick up her children.

Over the next few days, I spent quite a bit of time at the hospital. Momma was moved out of ICU and into a room that allowed visitors to stay longer. Because the hospital was relatively close to where I worked, I was able to go there on my lunch breaks. I also went back to the hospital after work. I sang to her, prayed over her, and talked with her during every visit. I also walked down the hospital corridors praying for the other patients who were on the same floor.

I had never seen anyone in a coma before. Momma looked so peaceful lying in the bed. A part of me wanted to believe that the doctors were wrong about her situation. Momma didn't look like she was in a coma. She appeared to be in a deep sleep and would wake up at any moment. I wasn't sure if she could hear me or even knew I was in the room, but I hoped she did.

I had informed my managers at work about my mom. They were very understanding and told me to let them know if I needed anything. I told them that I needed flexibility to leave work if an emergency arose.

Other members in the family took turns staying at the hospital. We made sure someone was always there in case Momma woke up. We also wanted to have someone there to talk with the doctors whenever they made rounds.

On March 12, my niece was staying at the hospital with Momma. She called me at work in great distress at 11:45 that morning and told me that a "code blue" had been called on my mom. I quickly informed my manager about the phone call and rushed to the hospital. When I got there, I found my niece in the hallway crying.

I tried to find out what was going on but was not able to get a clear understanding from her. I rushed to the room to learn that my mom had passed away at 12:05, shortly after my niece's call. I stood looking at Momma in disbelief. She had recovered many times before, and I expected her to recover this time, as well. I walked over to her with tears flowing and stroked her hair. I leaned over, kissed her on the forehead, and told her that I loved her. I began calling my other sisters and brothers to tell them the news. It was the hardest thing I had ever done.

After the death of my mom, Accuserlina showed up with her bag of charges. She tormented me with her usual messages, causing guilt and blame to rise to the surface again. "You should have gone to the hospital sooner. Why didn't you just take the children to the hospital when you first received the news that your mom had arrived instead of waiting? Maybe then she would have known you were there. How many times are you going to make the same mistake?"

Accuserlina used every weapon in her arsenal. "You should be ashamed of yourself. You didn't make time to be with your parents.

You weren't a good daughter. What makes you think you deserve to be a mother? You didn't call and visit your parents enough. You were too busy going to school, living your life, and being with your family. Your children will do the same to you."

Although my parents knew I would be there for them at the drop of a hat, thoughts entered my mind that maybe I didn't deserve children because I didn't visit as often as my parents wanted. I faced feelings of remorse, and knew I should have made coming home more often a higher priority. Was my not being able to conceive some form of punishment related to this? I struggled with the thought but also knew that Accuserlina could be quite convincing.

I felt so much anguish and regret. I loved, honored, and respected my parents. On both occasions of their deaths, I thought I had more time to be with them, but I hadn't. I hid my true feelings and pretended everything was fine, but it wasn't.

CHAPTER 11

Barren

For indeed the days are coming in which they will say,
"Blessed are the barren, wombs that never bore, and
breasts which never nursed!"
—LUKE 23:29, NEW KING JAMES VERSION

At the time of writing this chapter, I am fifty-three years old. I have been married twenty-one years and have never been pregnant. Medically speaking, I am categorized as being barren. According to the *Online Etymology Dictionary*, "barren" is defined as being "incapable of producing its kind." "Barren" is a biblical word that brought embarrassment and shame to not only the woman but also to her husband.

Why does infertility cause so much pain and embarrassment? Where and how did these feelings originate? More importantly, why do we allow it to still control our lives, especially in this day and age? Haven't we tormented ourselves long enough? I believe it is time for a change of mindset and the renewing of hope, faith, confidence, self-love, and the restoration of self-worth.

Barrenness carries a horrible implication of finality. It brings the message that life cannot be created because the womb is dead. The thought of not being able to have children made many women, including me, feel like less of a person. Being barren personally stripped me of my confidence, self-esteem, self-worth, and vitality. It created a stronghold over my life. As much as I resisted it, and despite my strong will, it captured me, and I became one of its emotional prisoners.

How did this happen? Why was the impact of infertility able to overpower me? It had affected not only my life but the lives of countless women before me. Is there an end to this vicious cycle, or will we forever allow ourselves to fall prey to infertility's torment? I wanted to trace back in time the negative images of barrenness to try to understand the true source of its strength.

I felt it was important to look at how barrenness affected women who lived long ago, and to understand why their inability to have children had such a damaging effect on them. Why did they feel disadvantaged? What did it do to their image and the image of their husbands? Why was having children so important, and why would not being able to have a child cause so much distress?

I did not know the answers that I would uncover but decided it was worth the time and effort to investigate. If I could get to the root of it, maybe I could help other women break free and rise above infertility's mental control. This would force the power of the emotional torment of infertility to finally and forever be diffused. As a part of my investigation, I wanted to seek answers from victims of times past. I would also tap in to my own experiences and understand why I was so emotionally impacted. My journey to find answers was about to begin.

Cursed. A failure. Defective. Rejected. Shameful. Disgraced. Worthless. These terms were associated with women of times past who could not conceive. Negative labels can be powerful. If an individual allows them to attach and accepts them as fact, it is difficult to remove them.

Having children was highly significant in biblical days. A man with a household of children, especially sons, was considered blessed, highly regarded, and respected in society. It was just the opposite for a household that did not have children. If a woman was barren, her husband was despised. They both were avoided and treated as outcasts.

This is demonstrated in the "Gospel of the Birth of Mary" in the Lost Books of the Bible. Mary's parents had problems conceiving. According to the scripture in this text, before her birth, Mary's father, Joachim, was ridiculed by the high priest because he did not have any children. The text reads as such:

> The blessed and ever glorious Virgin Mary, sprung from the royal race and family of David, was born in the city of Nazareth, and educated at Jerusalem, in the temple of the Lord. Her father's name was Joachim, and her mother's Anna. Their lives were plain and right in the sight of the Lord, pious and faultless before men. For they divided all their substance into three parts: one of which they devoted to the temple and officers of the temple; another they distributed among strangers, and persons in poor circumstances; and the third they reserved for themselves and the uses of their own family. In this manner they lived for about twenty years chastely, in the favor of God, and the esteem of men, without any children.
>
> But they vowed, if God should favor them with any issue, they would devote it to the service of the Lord on which account they went at every feast in the year to the temple of the Lord. And it came to pass, that when the feast of the dedication drew near, Joachim, with some others of his tribe, went up to Jerusalem, and at that time,

Issachar was high-priest; Who, when he saw Joachim along with the rest of his neighbours, bringing his offering, despised both him and his offerings, and asked him why he, who had no children, would presume to appear among those who had? Adding that his offerings could never be acceptable to God, who was judged by him unworthy to have children; the Scripture having said, cursed is everyone who shall not beget a male in Israel. He further said, that he ought first to be free from that curse by begetting some issue, and then come with his offerings into the presence of God.

But Joachim being much confounded with the shame of such reproach, retired to the shepherds, who were with the cattle in their pastures; For he was not inclined to return home, lest his neighbours, who were present and heard all this from the high-priest, should publicly reproach him in the same manner.

Not being able to conceive for twenty years must have been a heavy burden for Joachim and Anna. Her barrenness probably placed a tremendous amount of pressure on her and led to her husband's humiliation. I can imagine Anna hiding inside of her home, not wanting to be around the other women. It is likely she was concerned how they felt about her. This woman no doubt dreaded hearing the rude, thoughtless, and arrogant comments that were made and the scowling stares that were cast her way. She was likely pitied, ridiculed, disrespected, and frequently talked about.

I am sure Anna felt like a failure and had low self-esteem. She may have felt unattractive, useless, and unloved. In her mind, the one thing she was created for and commanded by God to do with her husband, to "be fruitful and multiply," was denied to her. How often did she watch the neighboring women who had conceived walk proudly with their enlarged bellies while smiling happily? Oh, how she envied them and prayed that one day her dream of having children would come so that her nightmare could finally end. The heartache she must have suffered.

One day Anna's prayer was answered. She conceived a daughter, whom they named Mary. Anna's shame and ridicule were finally lifted, and Joachim was accepted and no longer an outsider. Other women of biblical days, such as Sarah, Rebekah, Rachel, Hannah, the Shunamite woman, and the mother of Samson were all initially deemed as not able to have children.

It seemed as though a woman's social status was tied to her ability to conceive. The *Theological Dictionary of the Old Testament*, volume XI, states that the social position of a childless woman is revealed by the fact that she is despised and counted among the poor, the lowly, and the helpless. It also states that barrenness is the greatest disgrace that could befall a woman. But in Isaiah 54, the childless woman is told to fear not, because she will no longer live in shame. She is told to not be afraid because there is no more disgrace for her.

Yet the high priest told Joachim that he was not welcomed in the temple, nor would his offering be accepted, simply because his wife could not conceive. This type of treatment placed a huge burden and a great deal of pressure on the wife. It is understandable how women without children felt they lacked value and worth.

This attitude was the opposite toward women who were fertile. They were considered blessed and joyful. The more children they had, the more blessed they were considered to be. These women knew they were envied by the infertile wife. Some who were fruitful were unkind, arrogant, insensitive, and thoughtless. The Bible speaks of how Hannah was tormented by Peninnah, her husband Elkanah's second wife, because Peninnah consistently conceived while Hannah could not. This made Hannah weep bitterly (1Sam 1:10).

Rachel, the wife of Jacob, stated that if Jacob did not give her children, she wanted to die (Gen 30:1). That indeed was a desperate situation. She preferred death over being barren. Her sister Leah was fruitful and had several children, but for many years Rachel could not have a child. She allowed the people around her to label her as unworthy, which led her to repeat what they were speaking. The worst part was that she believed and accepted this as fact. Eventually, Rachel conceived and birthed a son, who was named Joseph. With this birth, she finally felt accepted and worthy. However, Rachel was never unworthy in God's eyes, nor was she considered unworthy in her husband's eyes.

Many women, even today, have bought into the idea that having children is the element that makes us special, while not being able to have them makes us less than average. Both of these situations are completely untrue. A woman is special and worthy whether she can conceive or not.

I can imagine that barren women of the long-ago past believed that their husbands could not love them if they didn't produce children. Perhaps they even perceived that the woman's life was not pleasing to God. Was a woman's unfruitful womb meant to bring shame upon her spouse's head and embarrassment to her household? Was this the ruling of God, or did people promote this way of thinking for their own purpose and power? God did not call barren women shameful or unworthy. I do not believe he intended women, past nor present, to feel this way.

How does the negative image of barrenness from long ago relate to the devaluing thoughts and emotions tied to infertility today? Life today is quite different, yet that same demoralizing spirit still exists in our society. Why? Is it possible that women in today's society who are challenged with infertility emotionally torment themselves because they consciously or subconsciously seek approval, validation, or acceptance, similar to the women of times past? I am not affirming that this is the reason for everyone, but it was a reason in my life.

Similar to Anna, I was barren for more than twenty years. The difference was that I never conceived. Since Anna was able to and I wasn't, does that mean that God's face was turned against me? No, it does not. What it does mean is that I played a part in creating that experience.

I needed to take ownership of what I had formed. I had walked under a cloud of condemnation related to not being able to have children. This was not the way it was meant to be. I operated as though I was broken, unworthy, and blemished. There was absolutely nothing I had done that should have caused me to feel ashamed or embarrassed.

The only power those thoughts and emotions had over me was the power I had given them. Understanding the history tied to the negative emotions and stigmas associated with infertility made a huge difference in how I had previously viewed myself. If the only power the negativity had was the power I had given it, that meant I could take that power back. This is exactly what I did. It is time to break the negative emotional spirit of infertility that has been tied to the lives of men and women. Hold your head up, take your power back, and know you are special and valued.

CHAPTER 12

Let's Adopt

I was chosen, I was wanted, I was cherished,
I grew in their hearts, I was the missing piece,
I was loved, I was adopted.

—UNKNOWN

After donating the fertility drugs to Dr. Kutteh's office, I had no idea what lay ahead for my family's future. I was doing my best to not be overtaken by the disappointment of no longer continuing fertility treatments but was having difficulty doing so. I did not talk much about it, but Chris noticed the distress I was experiencing by not being able to conceive. He was remarkably loving and supportive. His strength gave me confidence that everything would somehow work out.

One day, out of the blue, he said to me, "I believe the Lord wants us to adopt." I had been so consumed by trying to get pregnant that the thought of adopting had not entered my mind. The more I thought about it, the more peace I felt. Other than Chris's dad, we did not know anyone who had been adopted. We were not familiar with what was involved in the process or where to begin. I confided in a female friend at work about our interest in adopting, and she told us of an agency we could contact.

I called the adoption agency to inquire about their services. I informed the representative that my husband and I were interested in adopting a child within a specific age range. The representative explained the process. She said that Chris and I would need to successfully complete a training and preparation program prior to adopting. In January 2003, we received a letter from them that outlined the basic process requirements necessary to adopt. The letter also included information about their organization, frequently asked questions, and an adoption application.

Chris and I completed the application and were placed on the schedule to attend the next available training class. The class contained both married and unmarried individuals who either wanted to adopt or were interested in being foster parents. Everyone in attendance was excited and a little nervous. As an ice breaker, we all introduced ourselves by associating a word with the first letter of our names. I was Fun Frances, and my husband was Cool Chris.

We were each given a participant's handbook that outlined the purpose of the program and the expectations of each participant. During the next several weeks, my husband and I gained a wealth of information and an insight that forever changed our perspective. We understood that there was a great need for people who were willing to share their lives and homes, and open their hearts to children without families. I appreciated and respected the work that the adoption agency was doing in the community and their dedication to connect children with the right families.

Prior to starting this journey, Chris and I had no idea what the financial responsibility associated with adopting a child would be. Being an avid researcher, I began to search the internet in the hope of finding information that would give us insight. Much of the information was about applying for loans as a funding source for adoption. I learned that some banks offered loans up to twenty-five thousand dollars. My husband and I decided that we would not acquire any new debt as part of the process.

As I continued my internet investigation, I discovered that there were other financial aid options available for people looking to adopt. One option in particular caught my attention. I learned that many employers offered adoption expense programs as a benefit to their employees. I felt that this was the avenue Chris and I should take. With that in mind, I began to review my employer's benefits to determine if adoption assistance allowances were offered.

When I discovered that my company offered the benefits, I was elated. I could not wait to share the great news with Chris. Upon becoming more familiar with the company's adoption benefit plan, I became a little disheartened. I wasn't sure if we would be able to take advantage of it like I had hoped. The plan allowed for reimbursement of adoption expenses, but that meant we would have to pay for the expenses up front, just as with the insurance coverage for the IVF treatments a few months prior. History was repeating itself. The same financial roadblock that had hindered my husband and me from pursuing IVF treatments had reared its head again. Our savings had been used to purchase our home, and we weren't sure if there was enough left to cover adoption expenses.

Depending on the cost of the adoption, Chris and I would first have to get a loan and then apply for reimbursement. We had already decided that requesting a loan would not be a part of our adoption plan, so this posed a new problem. I searched for information in the plan that could provide other options but was not able to find anything. Suddenly, I had an idea.

What if the plan could be improved to more effectively benefit employees who used adoption to create their families? Maybe I could write and submit a proposal requesting a change in the company's adoption policy. It was worth trying. I felt good about this idea. The more I thought about it, the more it made sense. I made my decision and began examining the adoption policies of Fortune 100 and 500 companies.

After reviewing several policies, I began constructing a proposal to suggest changes that could be made to my employer's present adoption benefits. I was extremely excited to take on this project. Not only could it help my husband and I, but if it was accepted, it would give me the opportunity to help my fellow impacted colleagues in a special way. Additionally, it would give the company the opportunity to provide a greater benefit to its employees. It would be a win–win scenario.

I felt that a policy change would show a greater concern for the many employees who select adoption as an alternative way to create a family. At that time, adoptions were increasing in America. This reinforced my belief that the number of employees willing to consider adoption, especially those who had exhausted every possibility to conceive, could increase if my suggestions were incorporated. My recommendations would also assist in enhancing work-life balance. I put forth a great deal of time and effort to create my proposal. I shared the idea with my managers, and informed them of my plans.

I sent the draft document to them for review, and made a few changes based on their feedback. After my proposal was finished, it was time to present it to the company. My managers were supportive of my initiative, and connected me with someone to start the process. I sent an email introducing myself to the designated contact stating that I was in the process of adopting and had read through the company's adoption benefit plan to see what it covered. I mentioned that in my review, I saw areas in the adoption and parental leave section that could be improved to more effectively benefit employees who have chosen adoption to build their families. I attached a copy of my proposal and provided a brief overview of what it included.

My proposal contained three tables. The first compared the company's current policy to my suggested policy recommendations. One of the main components of my proposal was for the company to offer paid leave for adopting parents, much like the provisions offered to women going on maternity leave. Providing paid leave would give the adopting parent and the child time to bond as a family. Depending on the child's age, this is a crucial step in helping them to feel comfortable in their new environment.

The second table contained details of some of the adoption policy benefits offered at other companies. I provided the names of several companies that had taken the additional steps, including offering paid leave for adopting parents. These steps were necessary to promote the adoption process and to aid in providing support to those families. The third table outlined the various stakeholders and the potential benefits for the company, the employees, and the communities if the current policy were to be amended.

My proposal was sent to the department responsible for the adoption assistance plan. The feedback I received indicated that my suggestion had been miscommunicated and misunderstood. Because of this, my proposal was immediately denied. It looked like my idea had ended before it began. After receiving the news of the misunderstanding, I immediately responded to explain the purpose and intent of my suggestion.

I asked if the company could look at how the adoption plan had been written, see that there is a need, and find a way to change the policy so that need could be met. Over the next few months, I was involved in several conversations and email communications regarding my proposal. I was hopeful that it was gaining the right attention. I was also grateful that my concerns were getting heard. I had never taken on a venture of this type and was not sure what to expect.

There were occasions where I felt things were moving in the right direction. At other times, movement seemed to be completely stagnant. I continued to defend my idea because I knew it had merit and value.

Although I was uncertain if my proposal would be accepted, my husband and I continued progressing through the adoption training sessions. The outcome of the proposal would have no effect on our decision to bring a child into our home. There were several requirements that needed to be fulfilled in order to complete the training program. One in particular was quite memorable. Those who were interested in adopting were asked to create a presentation book.

The book was geared toward giving the reader a pictorial glimpse into the lives of adopting parents without revealing their names. Chris, Gabby and I worked on this project together. We purchased a photo album with a beautiful dahlia flower on the cover to house our family story. We went to several arts and crafts stores to find material that would make our book special, attractive, and welcoming. Chris is very artistic and had many creative ideas that made our album come to life. We had a lot of fun putting it together.

The first photo in the album was a wedding photo of Chris, Gabby and me. The caption beneath the photo was, "Hello, welcome to our family. This photograph reflects a wonderful and joyous day for us. It was the day that God first joined us together as a family. We are so glad that God decided to bless us with you."

Other photos represented captured memories of our lives, including vacations, holidays, graduations, and other special moments. We included a photo of our home and other family members, including grandparents, uncles, aunts, and cousins. We wanted to give an inside view of the love we have for family, our Christian faith, and the love that was waiting for the new child who would one day be in our home.

At the conclusion of the training program that September, the adoption agency presented my husband and me with certificates of completion. We were overjoyed. There were follow-up tasks that we needed to complete, including our home study, but we were one step closer to becoming adoptive parents. After all the forms and procedures were completed, Chris and I were approved to adopt. The next step was to be matched with a child.

Becoming qualified was one thing, but waiting for a child was another. The agency did not know how long it would take to find a child who fell within our adoption requirements. We were patient and willing to wait. Even if I conceived, we still would adopt. Chris and I wanted to not only bless a child who needed a family but also bless our family with the love of that child.

Although our plan was to adopt one child, I kept feeling there would be two. I felt it so deeply that I told Chris about it. I asked him how he felt if there were two children instead of one. At first, he was hesitant, but then he said that if the Lord had two children for us, we would adopt both of them.

Out of the blue, we received a call from the adoption agency saying that two children were available for adoption. They wanted to know if we were interested. At the time, the agency didn't have a lot of information about them. After they learned more, they informed us that they were two brothers in our age range. The agency representative wanted to know if they could bring the children into our home within the next couple of days, but my husband and I wanted to know something about the children before making that decision. We received some background information and spent time talking it over.

Our plans to bring one child into the family was quickly changing. We would never separate the brothers and would gladly welcome both. After we discussed it and consulted the Lord in prayer, we decided to meet the children. Prior to meeting them, I prayed for the children who were not yet mine. I asked God to watch over them and keep them safe. Although I had seen no more than a photograph of them, I was already starting to bond with them in spirit.

Arrangements were made for the date and place where we would meet the boys. Chris, Gabby, and I made preparations for the day, then drove to the designated location to meet them. They were ages two and four years old, a little older than their images in the photos. but were as cute and sweet as could be. The oldest was quiet but welcoming. The youngest was unsure of what was occurring.

We received the opportunity to bring the boys to our home for the weekend and spend time with them before making the decision to proceed. I was nervous but excited. I wanted everything to be perfect so the boys could have a great time. Chris and I made sure we had food they would like. He, Gabby, and I spent a lot of time laughing, playing, and making them feel comfortable. We all had such a wonderful time.

The following Monday, the adoption agency representative came to pick up the boys. I helped them to the car and promised that I would see them soon. After they left, I cried. I didn't want them to leave. After that, bringing the boys into our home permanently was an easy decision. We knew they were our children.

Chris and I talked it over with Gabby, who was ten years old and happy to be getting two brothers. We informed the adoption agency of our decision. A week later, the boys came to live with us. The adoption process would take several months to finalize. We now had to adjust and grow together as a family.

As part of the transition, my coworkers put together a baby shower for us. Chris, the boys, Gabby, and I sat at a special table in one of the company's conference rooms. I had attended many baby showers but had lost hope that one would ever be held in my honor. I will always remember the kindness my coworkers showed to us that day. I received cards of congratulations with kind sentiments and well wishes from many of them. I still have those cards today.

Bringing the boys into the family was a huge adjustment for everyone. We did as much as possible to help them feel at home. They were curious about everything and kept us on our feet. Chris and I bought bunk beds with matching sports-related comforters to help them settle in, and placed stuffed animals in their rooms. The bedroom ceiling was covered with illuminating stars that reflected at night. Their toy box was filled with fun toys and games.

We found a great home daycare that cared for other children their ages. The boys were learning new things every day and enjoyed attending. Chris and I learned that our youngest son was afraid of dogs. It took him a while to adjust to our Maltese, Angel. She was very friendly, playful, and happy to have new people in the house. Eventually, we couldn't keep them apart. Gabby was doing a fantastic job being a big sister.

Over the next few months, our new family settled in nicely. The boys were growing like weeds. They were getting taller, and both of them grew two clothing sizes. They had hearty appetites, a lot of energy, and were full of surprises. Both of them were happy and full of excitement but still shy and unsure of their new environment.

Chris and I constantly reminded them that our home was their home. We went to great lengths to let them know they were loved. Our sons were as much of a blessing to us as we were to them. They were both so precious and loveable. At bedtime, I tucked them in and made sure to either read a story or make up one. Sometimes I would sing to them as well.

Like I had with their sister, I gave the boys nicknames. The oldest was called Roddy and the youngest, Sugar Man. Roddy was quieter than his little brother. He had the cutest laugh that made us beam within. He loved getting new things. as it made him feel special. We bought him and his brother new suits for church. He loved wearing his, especially when we went to a restaurant. He would sit at the table smiling from ear to ear and being very careful not to drop food on it.

Roddy wasn't a big talker, but he loved hugs. I noticed that he was protective of his little brother; he appeared to believe that it was his responsibility to look out for Sugar Man. For example, on the day the boys came to live with us permanently, I announced to them that I would be cooking a special celebration dinner and asked what they wanted to eat. Roddy immediately said hamburgers, so I went to the store to buy groceries to honor that request. After parking the car, I immediately went to Roddy's side to get him out first before going to the other side for his brother. As soon as I closed his car door, he looked at me and said very seriously, "Where's my brother?" I smiled, led him to the other side of the car, opened the door, and showed him his brother. It touched my heart to see how close they were. It also amazed me that Roddy felt he needed to look out for his brother at such a young age.

Sugar Man, on the other hand, was spunky, outgoing, and surprisingly direct. He had large, inquisitive eyes and big cheeks, and was quite observant. Sugar Man loved attention and being held. He was comical and charismatic. Family meant a lot to him, and he had no problem letting anyone know how he felt on the subject.

I recall one day Sugar Man was watching cartoons in the living room with Roddy. My husband came into the room, gave me a hug, and then kissed me on the cheek. That caught Sugar Man's attention. He stopped what he was doing and said, "Stop kissing my momma. That's my momma." He was small but so serious. Chris and I thought it was funny, so he kissed me on the cheek again. Sugar Man looked at him, his jaws puffing in and out, and repeated, "That's my momma! Stop kissing my momma!" I laughed and said, "They're fighting over me." I walked over, picked him up, and gave him a big hug and a kiss on the check. Now, many years later, as a joke, Sugar Man will give me a hug for absolutely no reason in the presence of his dad. He first makes sure Chris is watching and then smiles and sticks out his tongue at him. The two of them are true characters.

Our sons had been living with us for several months by the time the adoption became final. The house was buzzing with excitement on adoption day. We were told when to be at the courthouse, and given basic information on what to expect. I felt so much pride and joy knowing that the boys were going to be a permanent part of our family. Afterward, we went to the adoption agency for a celebration party.

We celebrated with the agency staff, some family members, and a few friends. We were all smiles and laughter. Chris's dad shared his story about being adopted. One of the adoption agency representatives took our first family photo. They said that hundreds of siblings were separated each year because of the lack of family homes that could keep brothers and sisters from being divided. The agency expressed their gratitude in our willingness to keep the two brothers together.

Toward the end of the celebration, the adoption agency gave us a white candle symbolizing the day we became a family. They suggested that we light the candle each year on adoption day to honor this momentous date. After the celebration had concluded, we went home, where one more surprise was waiting.

My husband had hired a photographer to come to our house to take family photographs. We all wore similar outfits, and the photographer took our family photo, including our beloved Maltese, Angel. When we received the photograph package back, one of the pictures had an inscription that read, "And They Became One," along with the date of the adoption. People have said to me on countless occasions over the years how blessed our boys are to have been adopted. I always saw it differently. I knew how tremendously blessed we were that they were a part of our lives.

I never lost sight of the progress of the proposal I had submitted to my employer. After several months of going back and forth regarding my recommendations, I was informed that a final decision had been made. My proposal was denied. The adoption policy would not be changed. I was told that the company's benefits were externally competitive and provided the appropriate level of coverage. The news was disappointing, yet I remained positive. I believed wholeheartedly that my recommendation was valid. I felt that many would have benefited from my idea if it had been approved.

Ironically, two years after my suggestion was denied, the company decided that the adoption policy would be amended to offer paid leave for employees who were adopting children. By this time, Chris and I had finalized our adoption and were happily building our lives with our two new sons. Although my proposal had been refused two years prior, in the end, my dream had become a reality. Adopting employees would be able to have paid leave and time off to bond with their newly adopted children.

CHAPTER 13

Wearing the Mask

Behind every mask there is a face, and behind that a story.
—MARTY RUBIN

*J*essica, I thought with delight. *Her name will be Jessica. She will have my smile and high cheekbones and her dad's eyes and sense of humor. She will be beautiful, smart, and gentle yet strong, caring, loving, wise, and kind. Jessica will have a compassionate heart. She will go after her dreams and have a great life.* That's how I had imagined the daughter who would be conceived and born from the love Chris and I shared. I ended my daydream with great satisfaction.

Little had I known that this daydream was going to include many struggles. Since my diagnosis of severe endometriosis, and despite my repeated efforts to conceive, we had been down a long and disappointing turn of events. I had to move on with my life, and in the process, find some sense of peace and comfort. I was hurt, ashamed, envious, and angry. I still wore a mask to hide my true feelings from everyone I knew, including my husband. Doing so made matters worse, but it was my way to cope with the broken pieces in my world.

Even though we had three lovely children, it still hurt me to think that I would not pass on my blood lineage to future generations. It bothered me that I would not get the chance to experience life growing inside my body. It was upsetting to think that I wouldn't ever experience the mother-child bond that other mothers experienced with their newborns. I wouldn't get the chance to hear a baby say its first word or call loved ones to announce that my child had taken their first step.

I wasn't honest about my true feelings because I didn't want to be pitied for not being able to conceive. I didn't want others who were able to have children to feel awkward around me or make apologies because they could have children and I couldn't. I wanted people to think I was stronger than I actually was. I believed that the people in my life couldn't relate to why it hurt so much to not be able to get pregnant. It was easier to pretend than to admit the truth that my life wasn't as great as I wanted people to believe. Having a nice house, nice job, beautiful children, and a nice life doesn't mean one has a positive self-image. I attended church several times a week and served faithfully, yet I was broken inside, and no one knew it but me.

Under my mask, I was lost in a world of pain, envy, embarrassment, and resentment. It frustrated me to hear women who could have children say that they didn't want to have any more. Some even had surgeries to prevent them from having more children. I still longed to have what they were so willing to easily give up.

It saddened me to know that there were so many unwanted children who had been abandoned, neglected, mistreated, and unloved by women who seemingly had little or no appreciation for the precious gift they had brought into the world. It angered me each time these thoughts crossed my mind.

I needed to escape my feelings, but it was impossible to run away from myself. Since I didn't know how to move past the constant negative thoughts and emotions, I hoped that I could control them by pretending everything was fine. No one had to know what I was really feeling inside. I quietly picked up the invisible mask and slowly placed it on my face. I was smiling and laughing on the outside but was grimacing in heartbreak underneath.

I didn't need to wear the mask all the time. I only wore it during times of difficulty and disappointments. I put on the mask when one of my children didn't want to open up to me. I occasionally felt the need to put it on when hearing news of pregnancy and birth announcements from friends, family, or coworkers. "Congratulations!" I would remark, beaming brightly when I found out someone was having a baby.

I was genuinely happy for each person, but I could not deny my own discontent. The more it happened, the more envious I became, and the more I disguised my silent pain. It was like being a wall flower at a dance. You hope that someone will ask you to dance, but no one does. Instead, you watch everyone else enjoying themselves while no one knows you are there.

I was thirty-eight when we adopted our sons. We were overjoyed to have them in our family. Chris and I wanted to give them a loving environment. We sought out opportunities so each of our children could have productive futures. We wanted to enrich their lives and help them do well in life.

For a while, conceiving was no longer a priority for me. I had my three children and wasn't concerned about getting pregnant. I placed my time and attention on being with my three musketeers. Adjusting to life's changes was normal for our newly blended family. It took time for us to become familiar with each other's personalities and the additional responsibilities of having a larger family, but things were going well. Boys being boys, they were curious and sometimes mischievous, but that was to be expected.

Chris was a great dad. He taught them so many things. As they became older, he taught them how to ride bikes, mini motorcycles, and motorized scooters. He showed them how to play football and basketball. He even bought fishing gear and took the family to fishing rodeos. The boys had a special fondness for Gabby. They loved having a big sister who spent time with them.

The kids would make the most wonderful things in school. They would come home excited, bearing a school project that we would either put on the refrigerator or display somewhere else in the house. I still have almost everything in a large container designated for special family memories. I periodically dig through the container and reminisce of days long ago. The fondness of those precious memories always gives my heart a warm glow. As I think back, it was those special moments that helped me through some of the toughest times we faced as a family.

As the years passed and the children got older, our family started having challenges that opened the door to strife. Life became more complicated, and tension grew in the home. Gabby, Chris, and I began to have increased friction in our relationship. Gabby had become angry and rebellious toward us. It seemed as though everything was falling apart.

Chris and I loved each other dearly and would go above and beyond for one another, but we seemed to be moving in different directions. We began to disagree more frequently, especially when it came to the children. I felt he was too strict, and he thought I was too easygoing. Either way, we had to find a common ground and present a united front. Family life was getting stressful, and my reasons for wearing the mask were expanding. Something had to change.

I began to feel like a balloon caught in a breeze, just floating through life with no direction or purpose. I was merely existing from day to day. I didn't think I had any control over what happened in my life. I would wake up and prepare to face whatever occurred that day, but I was so focused on being the referee and trying to keep peace in the family that I was sacrificing my own peace.

I was giving so much of my time and energy to others that there was barely anything left for myself. How in the world did I get here? What happened to me? I had become invisible to myself and had lost touch with who I was. Many nights I would lie awake in bed and listen to the sound of the train in the distance. Even though I never wanted to leave, I would imagine myself on that train. I just needed to escape my reality, be free for a brief moment, and leave all of my cares and worries behind, even if it was only in my mind.

The older Gabby became, the more rebellious she became. When she entered her pre-teenage years, our relationship became even more strained; the closer I tried to get to her, the more she pushed me away. She even started combing her own hair because she no longer wanted me to do it. How could this be happening? I had been there for her for many years, helping her with homework, taking care of her when she was sick, and loving her the best way I knew how.

My daughter was slipping away from me. Our relationship was falling apart. It was bad enough to contend with fertility issues, but now my only daughter didn't want to spend time with me. I would lie in bed and sob heavily. I could not understand why everything had to be so difficult.

Chris tried his best to console me, but it didn't always work. He knew Gabby's rejection was deeply affecting me, but I didn't think he could fully understand the depth of my heartache. Gabby was his birth child, and I was her mom through marriage. Her natural mom was a part of her life, so Gabby gave me the impression that I wasn't needed or wanted. How could Chris possibly relate to what I was going through?

My husband sometimes found me crying after having an argument with Gabby and would do his best to comfort me. Then he would gently say, "Just let love rule." I did not want to hear that. I was doing my best to let love rule, and it wasn't working. But perhaps I only thought I was. In actuality, I was letting anger, hurt, frustration, disappointment, and irritation rule.

Life was much different when I was growing up. Children weren't outspoken with harsh words toward their parents. I was raised in an environment where children didn't argue or show any signs of disrespect to an adult, especially their parents. This was one of the core values Chris and I emphasized in our home. My parents had taught me this value, and I did my best to honor it.

I appreciated the sacrifices my parents made for me and my siblings. I didn't always agree with everything my mom and dad said and did, but I never let them know it. I wasn't the perfect daughter. Like many people, I made plenty of mistakes, but there were certain things we just didn't cross the line on. Showing a lack of respect was one of those things.

Seeing one of our children discard that value was a hard pill to swallow and could not be tolerated. If not corrected, this type of behavior could set the wrong example for the boys. I had to find a way to look past the things that Gabby was saying and doing. I had to be there for her even when I was hurting. I couldn't let my frustrations interfere with my desire to build a loving relationship with her.

I just wanted to love Gabby and have that love returned to me. I wanted us to be close, but that wasn't happening. Chris would tell me that no matter how she treated me, let love rule. His saying that would sometimes upset me, but deep in my heart, I knew he was right.

I thought it would be a good idea for Gabby to start spending quality time alone with her dad, so I suggested they start going on father-daughter dates. I planned special events for them and helped her choose outfits. It touched my heart to see her smile when they had their outings. Gabby seemed grateful for her special dates with her dad, and I began to see small improvements in our relationship, which made me very happy. We still had challenges, but I was hopeful that things would get better.

Out of the blue, one day Gabby announced that she wanted to go live with her birth mom. Our daughter had lived with Chris her entire life, and it really hurt him that she no longer wanted to be with us. But he wanted Gabby to be happy. After giving it a lot of consideration, he made the tough choice that no parent wants to make. He consented to Gabby's request to live with her mom. He thought that by letting her move out, perhaps the tension that had grown between the three of us would subside.

When she was fifteen years old, Gabby moved out of our home. It was difficult not seeing her every day. I missed her laughter, and the boys missed their big sister. Her leaving was a tough adjustment for us. Life was never the same. We were a family, but a big part was missing. I wore my mask more often. I was smiling on the outside but heartbroken underneath.

Gabby choosing to leave caused a huge empty space in our lives. I was upset that her leaving hurt her dad and her brothers. I was angry because she had left us . . . had left me. I understood her desire to experience living with her birth mom, but I didn't feel that her exhibitions of hostility and resentment should have been a part of the equation.

After Gabby moved out, I started having doubts about the bond and strength of our family. Even though the boys were still young, I feared that one day they would want to find and be with their birth parents. Would one or both of them choose to leave us as well? I thought that if I were able to conceive a child, I wouldn't have that problem. Maybe it wouldn't be so easy for a birth child to just walk away.

Hurt has a way of bringing out the most vulnerable and insecure parts of the heart. Being a parent can be tough; it doesn't matter whether it is a birth child, a stepchild, a foster child, or an adopted child. I was concerned about something that more than likely would never occur. My attention needed to be on the here and now instead of the "what may be one day."

My sons needed me more than ever. We were going to get through this difficulty together. A family is more than just DNA. Love has to be at the root of everything. Gabby choosing to move out didn't mean she didn't love us. I believe she was trying to fill a void in her own life. Being with her birth mom gave her the chance to do that.

Children will make decisions that we don't necessarily approve of or agree with, but sometimes we have to step aside and let them figure things out. I remember hearing a long time ago that if you love someone, set them free. If they return, they are yours to keep. I guess it was time to see if that was true. But how long would it take?

When people saw Chris and me with the boys, they often complimented their behavior, and constantly told us how much they looked like us. Chris and I knew there weren't any facial similarities, but it was always nice to hear. It especially made the boys feel special. They would grin shyly whenever they heard this compliment.

It would have been nice if my children had resembled me, but none of them carried my genes. Being adopted, they didn't have any of my biological makeup. It was sometimes challenging to figure the boys out because they didn't have our personalities or the character traits of anyone in our family line. It would have been easier to say, "Oh yeah, I used to do that," or "My uncle so-and-so is exactly like that." It was an interesting journey because we had no idea what to expect.

Another thing I didn't expect to occur were feelings coming alive that I had thought were buried. One day I woke up and realized that the yearning to conceive had resurfaced. I am not sure what stirred it up; maybe it was my cycle coming late. After all the years that had passed, I was right back where I had started. I found myself chasing the Fertility Fairy again.

There were times when I would search the internet for hours looking for a confirmation of my imagined, hopeful signs of pregnancy. I did this month after month, and was so disappointed whenever a pregnancy test was negative. After each negative result, I asked myself a series of questions: Did I perform the test correctly? Is the test faulty? Is that a faint double line? Could it be a positive result? Are my breasts looking fuller? They seem more sensitive than normal. I'm feeling more fatigue than normal. Why am I so moody? Maybe I am pregnant this time. And with those thoughts, I would hop back into my internet Ferrari and zoom down the interstate of pregnancy signs investigation.

The really sad part was that I secluded myself from my family to hide my disappointment, emptiness, sadness, and anguish. On many occasions, Chris didn't know that I had taken a pregnancy test. I kept everything to myself and chose to suffer alone. I was convinced that I was strong and could handle it, but it was foolish of me to try to handle it alone. I now cringe at the thought of the number of times I tormented myself this way.

To the outside world I seemed fine, but underneath the mask I wore every day, my heart was breaking. By the time I was forty-four, I had given up on any hope of becoming pregnant—or so I thought. I was in the peri-menopausal stage and having sporadic cycles. Even though they were not normal and were sometimes very light, I suddenly had hope. My imagination ran wild. I convinced myself that I was having pregnancy symptoms like the ones I had read on the internet.

I went as far as calculating a probable conception date. I even kept a daily record of every symptom I believed was related to my being pregnant. I didn't tell Chris about my suspicions, but I did confide in one of my sisters. My log captured details from the first day my cycle should have begun. My hope ended on day fifty-four when my cycle started. I took a pregnancy test as a precautionary measure just in case. Needless to say, it was negative. I was crushed. That was the last time I took one of those tests.

I can't count the number of times I was reminded that in the Bible, Sarah was able to conceive at the age of ninety. I know it was meant to be an encouragement, but it was not very comforting. I truly believe in miracles, but Sarah's case was much different from mine. It was a different time under different circumstances. If I conceived past age fifty, I would be grateful, knowing that God had a supernatural purpose for it.

After being married for almost fifteen years without conceiving, I thought that I had my emotions related to infertility under control. However, without warning, a boomerang hit me. I woke up early on the morning of August 12, 2013, with tears in my eyes, and wrote the following letter to God. I kept the letter and would like to share it here.

Dear God,

It's 6:40 am and I sit here in my bed, crying. I wonder why I was denied the blessing to conceive and bring forth a healthy child into the world. I wanted to have the experience of feeling life grow inside me. I wanted to know how it felt to be connected with a baby made with love. I wanted to raise that child and love that child and see that child grow up to be someone special. I try to let the feeling go, but it keeps coming back. Right now, it hurts to see other women have this privilege but know I haven't. I thank you for the children that I have been given. I thank you for the love I have for them and the love they have for me. I thank you for the millions of women in the world whom you have blessed to have children. Father, will I ever stop feeling this way? Will this longing ever go away? Thank you for drying my tears. I love you, Lord.

In Jesus' name, Amen

Letter writing was therapeutic for me. It gave me the chance to confront my issues and release the tension and hurt in my life. I don't know if the desire to bring forth life will ever completely go away; it has been such a huge part of my existence. I do know that the pain and sadness is no longer a part of my life. I had to find a way to break free from the anguish that I brought upon myself. I had to decide how long I was willing to pretend and conceal my true feelings. I needed to find my truth. I knew that when I found it, I would also find peace.

CHAPTER 14

Entering into the Light

We may encounter many defeats,
but we must not be defeated.
—MAYA ANGELOU

"Stick and stones may break my bones, but words will never hurt me." I said this phrase often when I was a child. I would say it to my siblings, as a joke to my friends, and to people I knew who didn't like me very much. I would say it while rocking my head from side to side. This was my way of letting them know that their words had no power over me.

Maybe, to a certain degree, there was truth to that phrase, but what I did not understand was that words are powerful. They are the primary way we create our lives and experiences. What is even more important to understand is that negative words spoken over us that are left unchecked can cause drastic harm to us, depending on who is saying them, their position of authority in our lives, and our own belief system.

Our own words and thoughts have the most power over us. They reflect what we believe about ourselves. If we are not careful, we can find ourselves viewing life as a victim and operating with a helpless, hopeless, and defeated mindset. Words spoken correctly can build a child up and help them to connect with their divine destiny. Words spoken incorrectly can rob that same child of their confidence and self-worth. A parent can speak hurtful words to a child who is desperately seeking their parent's approval, and can change the course of that child's life. Words can harm and words can heal. We make the decision on how we choose to use them.

René Descartes, who is known as the first modern philosopher, said, "I think, therefore I am." I have found this to be true. For a very long time, I allowed my own thoughts and words to strip me of my self-worth and self-esteem. Most importantly, I let my own fears, thoughts, and regrets torment me. I can be quite hard on myself, which can complicate situations in my life.

Our core thoughts are the building blocks for our belief system. It is vitally important to have a strong and positive belief system. Making the right kind of declarations over our lives can make a huge difference in our day-to-day experiences. If I understood then what I know now, I would have avoided a lot of pitfalls. I believe that one of the main roles of being a woman is to bring life into the world. When I discovered that I did not have the ability to conceive, I convinced myself that I was not as good as other women, that I was less of a person.

I didn't lose the gifts and talents I was born with. I was still a nurturer. I was still kind, smart, and intelligent. I was also a giving and helpful person. Amid all of my heartache, I was able to motivate, inspire, and encourage many people. The problem was that I was operating out of a partially filled container. I was determined to be strong because others depended on me. How could I admit what I was dealing with when I was supposed to motivate and encourage them? My thoughts were so draining that I wasn't able to replenish in proportion to what I was giving out.

Because I lacked the ability to conceive, I tried to compensate by portraying a picture-perfect image of myself, my marriage, and my family. I had a really good marriage, but it wasn't anywhere near perfect. There were flaws and cracks in certain areas, but I didn't want anyone to see them. I wanted my life to give hope to others, but it was I who had lost hope in myself. I didn't need someone born through my bloodline to prove that I was valuable and special. I was created with great value. But as a result of infertility, I became lost and forgot who I was.

When I was in my mid-thirties, I learned that my egg quality wasn't good and my reserves were low. I began to feel old and washed up. This weighed heavily on my mind. I am almost five years older than my husband, so knowing about my egg quality didn't help much. Although he didn't feel this way, I would sometimes think that maybe if he had married someone younger, he could have had the children he desired. I felt inadequate. I would eat a hearty breakfast of doubt and disappointment often. My confidence had diminished.

My infertility experiences were written with my thoughts, words, and beliefs. In retrospect, I believe the main reason I did not conceive, even before physical issues began to show up in my body, can be traced back to a thought I had in college. I wondered if I could have children. I pondered on that thought, not realizing that a powerful seed was being planted. As time passed, evidence to support that thought began to manifest.

Subsequently, fear, doubt, and the belief that I would never have children began to rise up in me even more. Hindering thoughts constantly lingered in my mind. Because they were so persistent, I soon began to wonder if there was truth to them. My thoughts told me I couldn't have children, so my words became, "I am barren. I won't be able to have a child." The more I thought it, the more it became real in my life.

Before I realized it, things were completely out of control. As much as I hate to admit it, to this very day, I have never conceived. I didn't fully comprehend it at the time, but life and death were truly in the power of my tongue. I thought, verbalized, and manifested one of my greatest fears, which ultimately became my reality.

Many words were associated with my inability to get pregnant. I experienced each of the feelings listed in table 2. Do you identify with any of them?

Table 2. Words with Power

Shame	Reproach	Pain
Anguish	Embarrassment	Anger
Resentment	Jealousy	Fear
Emptiness	Low self-esteem	Worthlessness
Condemnation	Blame	Sadness
Hopelessness	Distress	Loneliness
Heartache	Sorrow	Seclusion
Pretending	Lies	Defeat
Pride	Regret	Unattractiveness
Failure	Envy	Disappointment
Frustration	Doubt	Pity
Hurt	Moodiness	Judgmental
Irritation	Criticism	Bitterness
Guilt	Fatigue	Unforgiveness
Unapproved	Unaccepted	Not good enough

Although I wasn't able to get pregnant, I was blessed to have three beautiful children. As far as I was concerned, my family was complete. To my amazement, I still desired to get pregnant many years later.

After all those years with everything that had occurred in my life, why was getting pregnant still important to me? It wasn't about being pampered or getting a lot of attention. I just needed to feel complete. I spent so much of my adult life trying to prove myself to people. I wanted to prove I was a good wife, mother, friend, and sister. I even felt the need to prove to my siblings I was a good daughter to my parents.

I wanted my siblings, my in-laws, my children, and my husband to accept me for who I was. I always tried to do the right thing, but my well-meant intentions seemed to be misunderstood from time to time. I occasionally felt like an outsider. I was loved, but I felt disconnected from those who should have been closest to me.

I was so consumed by trying to be appreciated that I didn't realize I wasn't appreciating and loving myself. In my mind, having a baby would be a way of feeling connected to someone who was unbiased. This would give me that comforting closeness that seemed to be missing in my other relationships.

The bond between a mother and her baby is remarkable. There is such a strong connection that displays a pure and innocent love. A part of me believed that if I were able to conceive a child, I would finally receive the acceptance that I silently longed for. By conceiving and birthing a baby, I wouldn't have to prove myself to my child, compete for their love, or wonder if I was good enough. As the child grew inside me, a connection would form that could not be penetrated.

For years, I observed the bond that my daughter had with her biological mother. The love Gabby expressed to her was noticeably different from the love she showed toward me. They shared a special connection, one that I knew we would never have. I admit that I was envious, but I definitely understood. Their relationship was strong.

Sugar Man became interested in knowing more about his biological parents when he was in fourth or fifth grade. I openly shared information based on what I knew, the questions he asked, and his level of understanding. We had one picture of the boys' birth mother, which they could access at any given time. My husband and I were open to their asking questions about their biological family. Roddy, our oldest son, was preoccupied with other things and never seemed interested in hearing about them.

Regardless of his lack of interest, we made sure that both of them were present during the discussions. I tried not to show it, but having those conversations intimidated me. Despite how I felt, I did my best to make sure they had information about their past. The more we talked about it, the more I had to acknowledge that I had insecurities. *What if they wanted to find their biological parents? Suppose they preferred them over us?* The more I pondered on these types of thought, the more I questioned the strength of our family bond.

I loved my three children dearly and knew they loved me. Even so, I periodically struggled with the thought of one day being alone because they were not born from my womb. I was concerned that I would spend my life loving children who would one day leave me because I wasn't their birth parent. I thought that if I conceived a child, there wouldn't be a threat of that happening.

The reality of not being able to conceive had changed my perspective. It is amazing how circumstances can cause us to view life differently. When I was younger, it didn't matter that I didn't have children—until I discovered that I *couldn't* have children. Once upon a time, I did things to prevent conception. Later on, I found myself doing things to promote conception. It was remarkably ironic.

I didn't want people to know what I was experiencing or how I felt. I convinced myself I kept things hidden because I was a private person, but there was more to it than that. I was hesitant to speak openly because I felt others would either minimize the importance or wouldn't be able to relate to how it feels to not be able to conceive. How can a person truly understand unless they are able to view life through the eyes of someone who is trying to have a child but cannot?

I found myself trapped in the midst of a battle that I no longer wanted to be in. It was up to me to choose the best course for my life. It was time for me to change what I had been speaking over it. I had to learn to admit to myself that although my body was not necessarily functioning as God intended it to, I was still wonderfully and beautifully made. Yes, I was created to bring forth life, but I was not less worthy because I couldn't conceive. It didn't happen overnight, but I began to look at myself holistically and acknowledge that I was a strong and courageous human being.

I understood that I was not defined by my husband, my family, or my work relationships. I was also not defined by my reproductive organs or my inability to create life. I was able to realize that there was no reason for me to hide this part of myself. I did not need to be in fear of someone judging me. I no longer had to feel guilty or less of a person.

I came to the point where I decided enough was enough. I no longer listened to the deceptive thoughts that I wasn't good enough. I didn't need approval from the people in my life to be accepted. I had told myself that awful lie long enough. It was time for me to come out of the shadows and step into the light of recognizing who I was. I didn't need to receive consent to feel worthy. I was already accepted, worthy and valuable. I didn't need to conceive a child to feel blessed. I was already blessed. I became proud of myself and grateful for who I was.

After I truly understood this, I began to accept and learn to love myself. That is when the chains fell off and my healing started. I didn't need to conceive a child to feel closeness, love, and acceptance. Everything I truly needed was already there. I discovered that this kind of love had to be internal first. Then and only then I could truly appreciate the external love of those around me.

There are times when my mind tries to wander back to that area of self-doubt and of seeking people's approval. On those occasions, God gently reminds me that those whom I love do appreciate me, but it is His validation, love, and acceptance that matters the most.

Are you being challenged with low self-esteem, feelings of unworthiness, or thoughts that you have something to prove? If that is the case, know that you are not facing that battle alone. I am sharing the lessons I learned and some techniques that helped me. I hope that they help you, as well.

Find a quiet place where you won't be interrupted, then take time to consider and ponder the questions below. Be sure to journal your answers. Be honest with yourself, and listen closely for that still voice to guide you along the way.

Questions to Ponder

- What are your core thoughts and words related to having fertility challenges?

- How do they impact your life and those around you?

- What can you do to move past them?

- What are some steps you are willing to take to bring forth positive change in your circumstances?

It is important to watch your thoughts and words, for they truly have the power to create life. If you have challenges in this area, try the following techniques:

- Take control of negative thoughts by creating an atmosphere conducive to things that bring forth happiness. Listen to lighthearted music, watch or listen to something that inspires you, or perform a kind deed for someone.

- When you find yourself thinking negatively, do not speak the thoughts out loud. Instead, speak what you would like to occur instead of what you are thinking.

- If you find yourself in a sad or frustrated mood, take time to remember the blessings that you currently have in your life. Write down at least ten things you are grateful for and why you are grateful for them. Read and re-read the list, saying, "I am grateful for _____ because _____."

- Find a place where you can meditate without interruptions. Close your eyes. Breathe slowly, deeply, and purposefully. As your body begin to relax, say softly, "I am beautifully and wonderfully made. I was created to love and be loved. I am valuable, strong, caring, approved of, and accepted. A wonderful life is being created for me."

Pay attention to how you feel after you have done each technique. The more you do them, the stronger you will become.

CHAPTER 15

Let Love Rule

Take the first step in faith. You don't have to see
the whole staircase, just take the first step.
—MARTIN LUTHER KING JR.

The phrase "Let love rule" echoed in my mind. "No matter what happens or how you are treated, always let love rule." These were the words of wisdom Chris often said privately to me after Gabby and I had a confrontation. On certain occasions, this was not easy to do. I cried countless tears and felt great heartache knowing the only daughter I had, my daughter through marriage, had distanced herself from me.

Letting love rule didn't just apply to my relationship with my kids, however. It applied to every relationship I would encounter in life, including my marriage. It was to become the forefront of everything I did and the basis of every decision I would make. Sounds easy, right? Wrong.

The two greatest commandments in the Bible relate to love. Applying the principle of letting love rule when relationships are going great is a no brainer. It's a totally different story when you are in the midst of a battle. Notice I did not say in the midst of an argument; arguments are normally short lived. A battle is much longer.

A battle can cause a person to leave a marriage. It can make one want to give up on one's child. A battle can even make a person give up on life. These are situations where letting love rule is more difficult to apply. They can cause us to take a hard look at ourselves and determine how much that relationship really means to us.

I was going through a battle. As much as I hate to admit it, I sometimes wanted to give up on my relationship with Gabby, and there were times when I almost did. When we let love rule, we somehow find the strength to hold on. We have to hold on to the faith that things will get better. We believe for the best, even though the best is not what we are experiencing. Even so, still hold on.

Every once in a while, someone will come along and bring the words of encouragement we need to keep our fire of belief going. I can't count the number of parents who told Chris and me about their experiences with their child. They all gave the same ending to their story: things will get better when they get older. Those words were like a lighthouse in the midst of a dense fog. If it happened for them, maybe it would happen for us, too.

Applying the "let love rule" principle has helped me weather many storms. Here are some things that I have learned:

- Letting love rule involves looking deep within the person we are having conflicts with and finding the one thing in them that matters most to us. Perhaps that person has faults that are difficult to deal with but have a kind and loving heart. If that is the case, that is the part we keep before us. We focus on the good qualities they have and let that become our anchor.

- Letting love rule means letting go of any resentment and unforgiveness. We can't let love rule when we hold on to past or present hurts. In order to make this principle work, we must learn to forgive and release the hurt in our hearts. For some, especially depending on the severity of the situation, this can be extremely hard to do.

- Letting love rule helps us to ask for forgiveness, and forgiveness sets us free.

- Letting love rule can reduce the possibility of having challenges in the body. Relationships, especially those of a personal nature, correlate to matters of the heart. What effects the heart can ultimately affect our health if it is not resolved.

Letting love rule is a daily and never-ending process. As I continually search within my soul, I am finding and eliminating the residues of past hurts and insecurities. I lived with fatigue and emotional and physical pain due to hiding my true feelings inside. The hidden emotional heartache had manifested itself as pain in my knees and legs. I had no idea why I was feeling this way. I was in for a rude awakening.

There were occasions when the pain was so severe, I could barely walk. While at work, I would prop my feet up on top of an empty upside-down garbage can I kept under my desk. To keep the blood circulating in my legs, I would periodically get up and take a short walk. When I walked, I would put extra weight on my right leg to alleviate the pain on my left knee. Doing this shifted weight to my right leg, which caused it to hurt, as well.

The pain got so bad that I went to a specialist to determine the cause of it. After doing an X-ray and a thorough examination, the doctor informed me that I had a meniscus tear in my left knee. The doctor told me that I would need surgery to repair the tear. I scheduled the appointment for the procedure. After discussing it with my husband, I decided to wait a while before having the surgery.

I did not want to have surgery on my knee for various reasons. I needed a revelatory word to help me know what I should do. During my quiet time alone at home one morning, I presented the health challenge, and asked why I was having the pain and what I needed to do to be healed completely. As the words came into my spirit, I wrote them down.

This is the answer I received: "You are stressed, and it's causing the pain in your legs. You are trying to deal with everything on your own and will not allow anyone to help you. You cannot do this anymore without help. Let go of the pain and frustration that you are carrying (the heavy burden of being the one who has to do it all). There are others whom you can depend on to help you. Let them help you. Let go of the hurt and disappointment. Let go of the idea of betrayal. You can live again. You can be whole again. You can be the person you are supposed to be. Free your mind and your body. Learn to let go. The pain in your knees comes from stored stress in your body. Let go of the stress, and the pain will go away."

When I made it home from work that day, I soaked my legs in a warm Epsom salt bath. I then spoke out loud and released any negativity attached to me. Within a few days, I noticed that the pain had dramatically subsided. Since I was told by the doctor that there was a meniscus tear in my knee, I wore a knee brace to give it stability.

That was in September 2012. I no longer have pain in my knees or my legs. I did not have the knee surgery, either. I just needed to release the bottled-up stress, hurt, and disappointment that I had been holding on to. There is power in letting go.

Please keep in mind that letting love rule does not mean we

have to tolerate unkindness, manipulation, or mistreatment from anyone. It doesn't mean that we should let people take advantage of us. Letting love rule means having control over how we react and respond to relationship dilemmas. We can make a conscious choice to show kindness to those who are unkind to us. We can resist returning a rude response when someone is being rude to us.

If someone needs help and we have the capacity to help them, and if our heart is moved to do so, we can follow that lead. "Don't repay evil for evil. Don't snap back at those who say unkind things about you. Instead, pray for God's help for them, for we are to be kind to others, and God will bless us for it." (1 Peter 3:9, TLB).

I have had to apply the "let love rule" principle on many occasions with my husband, our three children, and others in my life. I have had to do the right thing even when wrong things were happening. I kept moving forward as best as I could. As the boys grew, they began to express their opinions in ways that didn't align with our family's philosophy. Chris and I began to see patterns that led us to believe challenges were to come.

I have to admit, being a mother was not what I had envisioned. There were many wonderful moments, but I thought it would be more rewarding and enjoyable. Sometimes I felt like a stranger in my own home. As my children got older, I wondered if any of them fully accepted me as their mother. They called me Mom, and they told me they loved me, but every once in a while, I felt a disconnection from them, like something was missing.

The only thing I knew to do was to let love rule. With this in mind, I set out to give them the best life I could. I made a fuss over them, supported, encouraged, and loved them with a sincere heart. I was determined to let love rule.

CHAPTER 16

A Real Woman

No one can make you feel inferior without your consent.
—ELEANOR ROOSEVELT

What traits does society require for a woman to be considered a "real woman"? The definition may vary depending on who you ask. Traits may include being strong, determined, intelligent, hardworking, dedicated, and successful. In my opinion, the biblical characteristics portrayed in Proverbs 31 are good examples. The *New International Version* reads:

> *A wife of noble character who can find? She is worth far more than rubies. Her husband has full confidence in her and lacks nothing of value. She brings him good, not harm, all the days of her life. . . . She is clothed with strength and dignity; she can laugh at the days to come. She speaks with wisdom, and faithful instruction is on her tongue. She watches over the affairs of her household and does not eat the bread of idleness.*

These qualities are not specific to being married. The important thing to note is that the woman described in these verses knows her value. She is honest, giving, and helpful to others. There is an attitude of confidence. She carries herself with respect. She is wise and prudent over the things under her care. She makes good decisions and handles business responsibly.

The definition that was used to describe a "real woman" when I was a young lady was quite different from the aforementioned list of traits. When I was nineteen years of age, I was involved in a conversation with a female acquaintance. During our chat, we started talking about kids. She suddenly asked me, "How many kids do you want?" Without missing a beat, I immediately responded, "I would like to have five children." She said, "You want five children? You're a real woman." *Really?* I thought to myself. *Wanting to have five children made me a real woman?* I beamed inside, believing that a desire such as this somehow made me special.

It never occurred to me to question how having a certain number of children would qualify me for this illustrious title. Perhaps the woman felt that going through labor that many times took great strength and endurance. She may have thought it was incredibly challenging to raise several children. I didn't ask her why she felt that way. As a matter of fact, I didn't really care. I just enjoyed the thought of one day being a real woman.

I knew several women who had multiple children. My mom and two of her sisters, who each had more than five, were among them. I loved and respected these three women. I knew they were real women, and if giving birth to five children was a qualification, I would be honored.

Life, with its sense of irony, did not allow me to birth five children, and not being able to conceive was a cruel joke to play. I often wondered, *What would that woman say if she knew my truth? Would she take away the title that she had so graciously bestowed upon me many years ago?* Was I no longer worthy of having it? Was I considered a failure when compared to the other women in my family? Tormenting thoughts entered my mind. *You don't have the five children you wanted. How are you going to have that many when you can't even conceive one? Where's that "real" woman you were supposed to be?* Accuserlina had struck again.

I made huge mistake when I gave my acquaintance permission to define, qualify, and categorize me. She knew nothing about the gifts and talents that were within me, nor did she know the goals I had set for my life. She wasn't familiar with my strengths, level of intelligence, or creativity. But she was not the one to blame. I had accepted her words as truth and wore them as though they were a medal of honor. I allowed something so inconsequential, in the grand scheme of life, to consume me. I also made the choice to ridicule myself because of it. I caused this unnecessary pain and suffering. I had to be the one to change it.

My being a real woman is not measured by the number of children I could bring into this world. It cannot be defined by others. As far as I am concerned, being a real woman is more about who I am inside. It is measured by my ability to sustain the positive force within, to overcome the challenges that life throws at me, and to rise above situations whether I can control them or not.

Life throws some of its hardest blows at women, and we yet continue to stand. We may be bruised, tattered, and fatigued, but we are still standing. Women, in general, are strong. We have a never-ending resilience and determination to keep moving forward. No matter how difficult a situation is, we somehow find the power to endure, even in the face of adversity. That is the definition of "real woman" that I live by each day.

CHAPTER 17

Rediscovering Me

You really have to look inside yourself and find your
own inner strength, and say, I'm proud of what I am
and who I am, and I'm just going to be myself.

–MARIAH CAREY

Who am I? What makes me special? What brings me joy?
What makes me want to wake up in the morning? What do
I care about? These are some of the questions I asked myself during
my journey to rediscover myself. Somewhere along the way, I had lost
touch with my true self, but I was determined to find her again. When
I did, I knew I would be a better version of myself, a woman who
would be stronger, wiser, more courageous, and more compassionate.

I needed to get back to being the person I was before infertility
entered into my life. I was not in a state of depression, but I *was*
consumed with the haunting thoughts of infertility. Something had
to change. *I* had to change.

After infertility entered into my life, I became exceptionally
private and protective of a fictitious image of a perfect marriage and
family. To the outside world, everything seemed fine for me, but deep

within, I finally had to admit that I was everything but fine. I had to rediscover Frances. I decided to perform an internal assessment of my character traits to help me get back to basics.

My true nature is comical, lighthearted, and a free spirit. I wasn't deterred by obstacles. Although I was unsure of the future, I was willing to step into unfamiliar territory. I believed in the abilities of others as much as I believed in my own. I inspired, encouraged, and brought hope and aspirations to those around me.

If someone said I couldn't accomplish something, I became determined to prove them wrong. I was calm in my spirit and comforting with my words. I walked with a quiet confidence and had stubborn, persistent faith. If someone I cared about was being mistreated or taken advantage of, like a mighty warrior, I came to their defense. My demeanor ranged from feisty, caring, determined, and bold to easygoing and playful. But as time passed, a fog appeared in my path and sent me off course. I needed to find a compass to guide me through the density and navigate me back home.

My first step was to make a list of the simple things that brought me happiness, even from when I was a young child. I included things like relaxing on a blanket in the warm sun, listening to the raindrops fall on a tin roof, and the smell of the earth after a Mississippi summer rain. These, among many other things, brought serenity and comfort to my life. I would find a quiet place where I would not be disturbed, and closing my eyes, I would think about the wholesome things that I loved.

Taking it one step further, I combined those thoughts with feelings. For example, I love watching butterflies. They are some of the most beautiful living creations in this world. Watching them float gave me a sense of peace and belonging. They made life seem pure and innocent. Butterflies reminded me to pay attention to and appreciate the wonderful things this world has to offer and to stay connected to nature. The same is true for rainbows and doves. They are constant reminders of peace, harmony, and love.

The chaos of infertility had caused me to forget this simple but necessary lesson. Remembering helped me to revisit a sacred part of my soul. This may seem odd or unnecessary, but if you have ever lost touch with who you are and found yourself behaving as someone you were not meant to be, it will make complete sense.

I expanded and expounded on several of the character traits that made me special and the things in life that gave me joy. As I recorded each item, I noticed my attitude shift in a positive direction. The more I wrote about and embraced a fond memory, the better I felt. I became so filled up that there was not any room left for negativity. That which had held me back was losing its effect.

A new hope entered into my heart in the form of making a simple but important decision. I chose to not be defined by my circumstances nor allow my happiness to depend on the ability to get pregnant. I chose to not allow any diminishing negative thoughts or beliefs that I had previously entertained control me. My attitude toward life would not be predicated on my being the ideal mother. My existence was much more than getting pregnant or having children. I took a hard look at my life and had to be willing to confront my fears and the lies that had mocked me for numerous years.

An amazing change burst forth during this rediscovery journey. I no longer carried the burden of being unable to conceive and having a perfect family image. I had no need to hide behind a mask because my mind had been set free from the bondage I had created. I was no longer ashamed of my circumstances nor critical of myself. As I removed the mask, I was able to see my true inner beauty.

The pain I had felt for many years began to go away. I was no longer tormented by negative feelings and self-destructive thoughts. I stopped being a victim of insecurity and discouragement. Although the desire to conceive hadn't disappeared, the inability to do so no longer had power over me. I regained strength and courage within. I found the confidence and desire to openly tell others about the emotional pain I had endured as a result of my inability to get pregnant.

I began to walk and live in the light of this truth. Peace, happiness, joy, acceptance, and self-esteem returned. Seclusion, self-pity, blame, shame, embarrassment, and the need for acceptance disappeared. I recognized that my inability to conceive, and the challenges I had experienced, had a greater purpose. When I realized this, life became more meaningful. As long as I was tied to what I didn't have, the pain, negativity, and emotional stigmas remained. As soon as I was willing to let it go, my heart, which was once heavy, became full of life again. I had taken the focus off of myself and placed it on giving back to others. That, in and of itself, is true healing power. Taking those steps was instrumental to my being free.

Questions to Ponder

What are some character traits about yourself that you have lost touch with as a result of being affected by infertility?

What are some things you enjoy doing that you have stopped doing due to infertility?

How has stopping those things impacted your life?

What are some personal and meaningful things that used to bring you serenity that you no longer notice?

If your challenges with infertility have completely overwhelmed you, you may not be operating like your normal self. If that is the case, you can benefit from these techniques:

- Become reacquainted with yourself by making a list of your character traits before infertility entered your life. Take note of things you liked about yourself that you no longer exhibit.

- Take your mind back to days of childlike innocence. Find a quiet spot where you won't be disturbed, and write down as many things as you can remember that brought you happiness. Be willing to go back to when you were very young. No matter how simple or silly it may seem, create an atmosphere of wholesomeness.

Review the list from the second technique, then pick one item, close your eyes, and see yourself doing that particular thing. Focus on how it makes you feel. If it makes you smile, laugh, hum, or sing softly, give in and go with it. Do this with as many of the items that time allows.

Take note of how you feel after completing the exercise.

CHAPTER 18

Breakthrough

If you want to see the sunshine,
you have to weather the storm.
—FRANK LANE

How long is long enough? What causes a person to finally decide that it is time to make a change? For many years I had given my time, attention, and energy to a way of life that was not in alignment with the dreams of building a family I had when I was younger. I lived in fear, shame, and doubt because I could not bring forth life in my body, like many other women did. The bigger question was, why did I allow this to continue?

Throughout this ordeal, I dealt with a lot of turmoil, confusion, emotional stigma, and heartache. I thought having children was something that I could control, but I ultimately had to accept that this was completely out of my control. Yes, I could have fertility treatments. Yes, I could have surgeries to help resolve some of the issues that prevented me from conceiving, but I could not make conception happen no matter how much I wanted it or how much I tried. There had to be a reason I was dealing with this, but nothing made sense to me. It just did not add up.

The very idea of being diagnosed with infertility hurt unlike anything I had ever experienced. I kept it a well-hidden secret from everyone I knew. The silent tears I cried were those of a person in mourning.

I frequently brought flowers to the grave of an empty womb, knowing that life would never form or grow there. Those who knew me saw me smile, but if they had looked closer, perhaps they would have seen the revealed truth in the sadness in my eyes. They may have seen that the smile I displayed was not always genuine. I was hurting, and no one knew the depth of that pain but me. It wasn't their fault. I had become the great pretender. I thought it made me strong, but it had made me vulnerable to the attacks of the enemy against my mind.

I didn't always feel accepted or good enough, so I spent a great deal of time trying to prove I was a good wife, mother, and daughter. I believed that if I accomplished this, the people in my life would give me the acceptance and approval I thought I needed. I was focused on how I thought others viewed me. I didn't know how to love and value myself.

I allowed the negativity of infertility to consume me to the point that I wasn't appreciating the blessings I had in my life. If, in God's eyes, I was fearfully and wonderfully made (Psalms 139:14 NIV), why did I cast shame upon myself? Why did I call myself damaged goods? Why did I label myself a failure? I was so absorbed in the pain of not being able to conceive, I forgot about the gifts and qualities that were within me.

I had allowed the thoughts of being barren rob me of my joy, peace, and true essence. If you are finding yourself doing this, wake up. Wake up right now and claim your life back. I didn't think I could talk openly about my feelings because most of the people I knew didn't know what if felt like to be barren. I made the drastic mistake of allowing infertility to define who I was.

I had to make a decision to no longer let something I couldn't control have power over my life. I refused to allow the heartache of not being able to conceive be the final chapter in my life. Like a person who fervently searches the sky for a break in the clouds after a heavy storm, I watched the clouds that hovered over my heart, waiting for the sun to break forth. Surely that day would come. But when? I was ready for the change and would welcome it with open arms. I prepared for it by searching within myself and acknowledging the mistakes I had made.

Suddenly, that day finally arrived. I awoke from the nightmare of my own torturing thoughts and false beliefs. I rose above the ashes of despair to recognize who I was and the power and strength that dwelled within me. I was released from the fears and emotions that had imprisoned me. It was time to do some final house cleaning.

I asked myself a few thought-provoking questions. Why did I believe I was damaged goods? What led me to believe that not being able to conceive made me less of a woman? Why did I feel it was better to hide the truth about the pain of not being able to get pregnant? Why did I feel the need to be ashamed? I realized there was not a need for any of those things.

I changed the way I thought about myself. I let go of the anger and all of the ugly, cruel accusations that had entered my mind. I accepted that I was worthy and valuable despite being infertile. My reproductive organs didn't function as designed, but I am much more than biology.

Another important piece of my evolution was in the area of forgiveness of self. Forgiveness is a true healing power. I had to forgive myself for opening the door to anger, resentment, self-ridicule, and condemnation for not being able to birth children. I had to forgive myself for being annoyed with women who could conceive. After

I forgave myself, it didn't matter who I thought accepted or didn't accept me. The real key was that I accepted myself. It was liberating.

Coming out of the valley of infertility wasn't easy. The good news is, because it was possible for me, it is possible for you. Just as I did, you will have to choose to let go and move forward.

As I changed the way I thought and felt about myself, I began to build a new reality. With that new reality came a sense of freedom. No more masks for me. I no longer wept for the child I couldn't conceive. The thoughts and feelings of unworthiness, shame, and heartache suddenly vanished. It no longer bothered me to see a pregnant woman glowing with joy and excitement. I was able to become even more appreciative for those who had received what I had desperately wanted but could not obtain.

I came to understand that children were not a part of my family just to raise and nurture. They are there to help me become a better version of myself. Children helped me to discover the areas in my life that needed pruning and reforming. Through children I have learned patience, compassion, love, and selflessness. They help me also recognize those emotions that I have not yet mastered. From this perspective, I see that I wasn't required to birth children in order receive these gifts. It simply took having children in my life for me to learn one of the greatest lessons of life.

What intrigues me is that I didn't see how anything good could come from my years of sorrow. All I could see was me and my pain. Never did I imagine that I would be sharing this intimate part of my life with others. Yet here I am. The changes I made in my life were intentional. I had taken a long look at myself and knew that the person I saw was not the person I was meant to be.

I had fallen and no one was responsible for helping me to get up but me. The people in my life could be there as support, but I had to make the decision to change. It was also my responsibility to follow through with it. Breakthrough is possible for every person reading these words. I believe that for you.

Questions to Ponder

- If you have kept your infertility challenges a secret, what concerns you the most about people learning about it?
- Why do you feel this way?
- What are some things related to infertility you believe you can control? What do you believe you cannot control?
- The negative emotions associated with infertility can be overwhelming at times. What are the top five emotions you would like to overcome?

The next time you find yourself affected by unwanted emotions, fertility related or otherwise, do the exercises below.

Exercise 1: Emotions Self-Awareness Assessment

The moment you feel a negative shift in your emotions, ask yourself the following questions:

- What just occurred that has caused me to feel like this?
- Do I want to feel this way?
- If the answer is no, then how do I want to feel?

Direct your mind to a thought or memory that will bring you peace or laughter. You may need to do this more than once, but be persistent. Be mindful that it takes little effort for negative thoughts to enter the mind and change your mood. You have to be intentional to make a positive shift in your thoughts.

A good way to navigate through negative feelings is to search within yourself to understand and address their root cause. After doing so, you will more easily be able to determine the next step in moving forward.

Exercise 2: Emotional Perspective

Use the chart in table 3 to capture any negative emotions you experience throughout your day. This will help you to become aware of how your emotions impact the way you view situations in a particular moment. The emotion doesn't have to be related to infertility. This will work with any scenario.

List an emotion you are experiencing, define the reason for it, and then record what would happen if you didn't feel that way. Let the answers in the third column be your primary focus to help you to shift your energy. The goal is to quiet your spirit so you can make an intentional conscious choice on how you should respond to a situation. Doing this will shift your energy to a positive nature. I have provided a couple of examples for you.

Table 3. Recognize and Shift Your Negative Emotions

Emotion	Reason	What if I didn't feel this way?
Discouraged	My friends and family have children, but I do not.	I would be more excited about the wonderful things I already have in my life and focus on the things I can control.
Anxiety	Started a new project at work and have a tight deadline	I could work with confidence knowing that I will do a great job and complete the assignment on time.

Please note, there may be occasions when you don't know what caused the negative feeling. If that is the case, sit quietly, close your eyes, and ask yourself, "Where did this feeling come from?" Wait a few minutes to see if an answer surfaces. Then state, "This is not the way I want to feel." Immediately tell the feeling to leave and to go back to from whence it came.

As a way to continue living a breakthrough existence, surround yourself with phrases that will inspire a positive outlook. Doing so will be a constant reminder of who you are and how you should be. Consciously avoid saying negative words you know you commonly speak.

In my home I have framed phrases such as "I am worthy" and "Happy thoughts, happy life." These phrases have deep meaning for me because at one time I felt I was unworthy, and on numerous occasions I did not have happy thoughts. I specifically chose phrases that would counter the thoughts I had entertained and believed for many years.

If you choose to follow this technique, be sure to find words or phrases that are meaningful to you based on your specific experiences. Every time you read a phrase, take a moment to pause and emotionally connect with it.

Even though you may struggle with negative emotions, talk as if you are already free from them. You don't have to wait until you fully see your breakthrough. Most times you will have to believe by faith before you actually see the results of your expectations.

CHAPTER 19

A Purpose and a Plan

As I look back on my life, I realize that every time I thought
I was being rejected from something good, I was actually
being redirected to something better.

—DR. STEVE MARABOLI

Life is filled with lessons that are waiting to be discovered. Each lesson we learn can build a multitude of qualities. Some lessons are tougher than others, but I believe those are the ones we should value the most. Through them, who we are and what we can become is revealed. Fighters, champions, leaders, nurturers, healers, and helpers emerge from the flames of adversity. This is the time when purpose and destiny come forth.

Once upon a time there was a young girl who had dreams of being the mother of five children. That desire was triggered by the love and example set by her parents. She did not know that life would throw a curve ball that caused her path to drastically change. She was diagnosed with infertility and was never able to conceive a child. For many years she suffered in silence, not realizing that something far greater was being created. Every heartache and tear she shed was tied to a purpose and a plan. She only needed to recognize it and accept the new direction life was taking her in.

This is the story of my life. I went through many painful infertility experiences, but my pain was not in vain. In the midst of it, purpose was born. I didn't know that I was in the process of being awakened and transformed, nor that I was being trained to help and encourage others through the emotional side of their infertility experiences. Everything I went through finally made sense.

My journey was not just about me. Although I endured infertility challenges, I never dreamed that they would be used in such a profound way. I was not taught about having a purpose and a destiny when I was growing up. These were not part of the conversations in my home. As an adult, I came to understand that I was dissatisfied with my life partly because I did not realize I had a divine purpose.

As I traveled the path of rediscovery, I learned that my life had a purpose that was bigger than my wants, needs, and existence. It was more than having a family. I realized I had an important assignment on the Earth. Although I didn't know all of the details, I knew it would begin to unfold. I was meant to help people in a very special way.

I was created to encourage and inspire others to become a better version of themselves. This awareness helped me to take the focus off of myself and place it on those I was called to help. With that perspective, my personal concerns were not as dramatic as I thought they were. The challenges I faced with infertility were the key to opening the locked door that had been concealed from me. I now saw things in a different light.

I had connected my life with purpose and destiny, allowing me to understand who I was meant to become. I felt whole and was excited about the possibilities for my future. A paradigm shift had occurred, placing me on a new journey. As I moved along this path, I knew more about myself and that the things before me would be revealed.

I had been emotionally stuck but became willing and determined to take the necessary steps to move forward. It didn't happen overnight, but it did happen. I had to change my thinking and reacquaint myself with the woman I was created to be. That woman is special and has tremendous value. Having the ability to conceive was not what was going to make me special, nor was bringing life into the world. It definitely was not what made me a "real" woman, although my inner thoughts convinced me for several years that it would.

I had lost sight of these important facts, but once I regained them, life became more rewarding. I remembered that every moment of each day in some way contained a miracle. When I was battling with infertility, I sometimes missed appreciating the miracles in my life because I was too consumed with focusing on what I considered to be one of the biggest of them all. Now I can say that every wonder of life, regardless of the size, is of great significance.

I am filled with new hope and optimism. My eyes have been opened, and I have found a greater appreciation of the wonderful blessings that are in my life. I understand why it is important to be thankful for all things. I realize that everything has a purpose and a plan. Even the things that are hurtful can be used to help strengthen someone else. I know what it means to go through infertility. That is why I am here as part of a support system for others.

CHAPTER 20

Looking Forward

Open your eyes to the beauty around you, open your
mind to the wonders of life, open your heart to those
who love you, and always be true to yourself.

—MAYA ANGELOU

Infertility was a difficult journey for me. Not just because I wasn't
able to conceive but because of the devaluing choices I made. I
allowed myself to be embarrassed by events out of my control, and
lost touch with the person I was chosen to be. I forgot that I was
blessed long before I experienced barrenness. I resolved to hide
behind a mask of pain, loneliness, and disappointment rather than
embrace and accept the idea that I did not lose importance just
because I couldn't bear children.

I want anyone who reads my story to make sure you do not allow
the inability to create life to steal the beauty and power of who you
are. Don't let it cause you to be uncomfortable, bitter, resentful, or
angry.

I was diagnosed with infertility more than twenty years ago, but
my thoughts and words created a situation that produced barrenness

in my womb. If I had understood the ramifications of what I was doing sooner, it is possible that I could have reversed the negative creation process that prevented me from conceiving.

If you have been doing this, make the choice to stop. Recognize that consistent negative thoughts and words can bring unwanted things into your life. You must be adamant about moving away from the things you want to discard.

One of the greatest lessons I have learned during my infertility journey is to release what is not beneficial for me. Keeping my eyes looking forward, I have been able to leave behind the hurtful thoughts, feelings, and letdowns I had contended with. I ceased bringing the garbage of yesterday into the beauty of my new day. This simple adjustment in my attitude empowered me to make better choices thereafter. As it related to infertility, I had the tendency to embrace ideologies that were not profitable for my self-esteem, which made it difficult for me to move forward. This caused me to remain stuck in an existence that I didn't want to be in.

Keep in mind that your thoughts and words are some of the most powerful tools in your arsenal. You can use them in a positive manner, or you can use them negatively. For example, if a person thinks that not being able to have children makes them worthless and speaks that affirmation with intense emotions, then these beliefs and feelings of worthlessness will begin to gravitate toward them. But if that same individual shifts their mindset, they will begin to understand that fertility problems are not synonymous with defeat. Those feelings and beliefs will dissipate, causing the individual to no longer accept thoughts of worthlessness even if they continue to have challenges conceiving.

During my journey through infertility, I have met women who avoid baby showers like the plague. They refuse to have anything to do with them. I get it, and it is completely understandable why they feel this way. Being invited to a baby shower is a reminder of what they don't have. For some, it is awkward and uncomfortable. They feel like they are caught between a rock and a hard place. They don't want to disappoint the person who invited them, but they also don't want to have to pretend to be happy about the occasion when a part of them is not.

When you think of baby showers as a negative event and are frustrated by them, you begin to push your desire away. I would like to bring forth a perspective that will perhaps help you to look at this situation differently. Why not look at being invited to baby showers as life's way of showing you what you could have? You can project into your heart that you want children and that you are being placed in situations where you are coming into contact with people who have received what you desire. You may not realize it, but you are then drawing pregnancy to yourself.

Here is an example I like to use. Have you ever thought about getting a particular type of vehicle or are going to purchase it? Let's use in this example a Ford F-150. As soon as you start seriously talking about it or are looking to buy one, you suddenly start seeing that truck everywhere. You may even see the exact body style and color you want. Prior to this, you had never noticed the Ford F-150. Once you decide you want one, you see them everywhere you go. As a game, you may start counting each one you see. That is because you have attracted that vehicle to you. Believe me, it is not just a coincidence. Signs are all around us that we often miss because we are focused on other things.

I believe that when you are being invited to baby showers, you are attracting a baby to you. You probably don't realize it because you are focused on the grief of not being able to have a child. Instead of looking at it as a heartache and a reminder of what you don't have, look at it as, "I am drawing to myself what I want." In essence, that is exactly what you are doing. Don't fight what life is trying to share with you. It is trying to give you a message of hope, encouragement, and possibility.

When I was trying to get pregnant, I attended baby showers as often as I could. Each time I went shopping for a gift, I put my heart into it. I bought the cutest outfits and selected heartfelt cards. I did it as though I were buying a gift for my own child. I sowed seeds for what I believed was going to happen in my life.

Although I never got pregnant, I was able to finally attend a baby shower that was given in my honor. When my coworkers held an adoption celebration baby shower for us after we adopted our sons, I received an abundance compared to what I had given out, and not just in receiving gifts for the children. The joy and happiness I received on that day will always stay with me.

I finally began to make the connection to what life was trying to show me during the period of my life when I couldn't get pregnant. My inability to conceive was in no way intended for me to fall prey to despair and self-criticism. Although I was faced with a difficulty in my body, it was never meant for me to lose sight of my value. I stopped thinking of myself as damaged goods. I stopped viewing myself as someone who was inferior to women who could have children.

I started seeing myself as I truly am, which is someone who has a big heart for people and who loves children. That is the part of me that I embrace the most. Even though my children are now adults and I am no longer in the season for having children, I still buy baby shower gifts with the same love and enthusiasm as I did in times past. I enjoy giving, especially to first-time mothers. I use baby showers as opportunities to sow seeds of love and kindness into the life of a new family.

Creating life is a beautiful thing. Women who are able to birth children are blessed, but it is not the only thing that makes us special.

I am not saying it is wrong to feel sad, angry, or any other emotion that accompanies having fertility challenges. I am saying to not let it consume you. Don't allow words spoken by others who may not know why you haven't had children dishearten you or cause you to think less of yourself. Look forward to a brighter future.

This story is about my life, what I went through, the mistakes I made, and the enlightenment I received. It is meant to be an aide to help you get past the emotional hurdles you are encountering throughout your infertility journey. I wrote it for all of the women and men who have suffered in silence while battling challenges to building their families. I wrote it for all of the relationships that were destroyed, or nearly destroyed, because there were difficulties in having children.

Maybe you are hurting because you so badly want a child but nothing you have tried has worked. I know that the stress of it all can seem more than you can bear. If this is your story, too, know that you can find the strength to carry on. You are not alone. Hurting hearts can be healed.

You don't have to go through your entire life feeling that life is over if you don't have a child. That is nowhere near the truth. There are options available. Some people who cannot conceive may decide to be child free. It is completely okay if that choice feels right. Some may decide to adopt, while others do not want to pursue adoption. That is okay, as well. Regardless of what you decide, the most important thing is to free yourself from the tormenting thoughts that come and cause sorrow. Please remember that having a child does not make you more of a woman (or man). Similarly, not having a child does not make you less of a woman (or man).

You are a wonderful, powerful, special, and important person. Don't let the fact that a part of your body does not work as you want it to rob you of your zeal for life. I learned this lesson the hard way.

In time, I came to realize and accept that a nonfunctioning body part did not cause a deficit in who I am as an individual. Avoid letting it change who you are and how you view yourself.

I am considered to be barren, but because of the revelation I walk in every day, that description no longer causes me shame. I have overcome the emotional stigmas of infertility. I am at peace with not being able to conceive. I am free. It is all about having the right mindset. The thoughts, feelings, and emotions that once held me bound are no longer able to disempower me. This can be true for you as well.

Emotional freedom is available for anyone. Looking forward is a huge step toward moving forward and obtaining that freedom. I was trapped in my emotions for a long time. It does not have to be this way for you. There is an opportunity to make a positive change in your life starting today.

This is a choice that only you can make. Are you ready and willing to make the necessary change? I believe you are. If that is the case, start by repeating the following affirmations. When you first start, the words may express the total opposite of what you feel, but don't let that deter you. Continue each day, as often as you can, and like me, you will see a change in how you think and feel.

I am strong. I am courageous. I am valuable.

I am special. I am confident. I am worthy.

I am free from all negative emotions and stigmas associated with infertility.

I am not ashamed or embarrassed by my circumstances related to fertility.

I am looking forward so I can move forward.

I am at peace with infertility.

Even today, I sometimes wonder what my child would look like if I had been able to conceive one. I imagine which of my or my husband's traits would have been passed down to that child. From time to time I still feel a longing to know what it would have felt like to have a child growing inside of me. I am not sure if that longing will ever completely go away. On the other hand, I am not sure I want it to.

It no longer bothers me that I wasn't able to get pregnant. I was able to accept that this was a part of my life and existence. No doubt about it, I love my three children with all my heart, just as though I had birthed them into this world. It took me a long time to get past infertility's negative stigmas and emotions, because I was trying to do it on my own. The weight became so heavy, but with God's help, I was able to withstand it.

As I look back over my life, I acknowledge that my trying to handle everything on my own had a reason. I believe that I was meant to go through the things I experienced exactly as they occurred. If it had not happened in the manner it did, there likely would have been limitations on my ability to help others in this area of life. I was able to release my feelings and speak openly about what had transpired in my life. I no longer have the perspective of a victim but the vigor and passion of a victorious person.

Someone recently asked me how long my infertility journey lasted. Since I was never able to conceive, I would say that after more than twenty years, my journey still continues. Although I live it every day, I have taken on a new perspective. My life has a deeper meaning because I took the focus off of myself and put it on others. I want to help people who are facing what I had faced. I am now exceedingly grateful for the challenges I encountered. They have made me a better person. I am hopeful that my story will help you in your journey.

The emotional scars associated with infertility can make a person lose a huge part of themselves. With strength, support, determination, and a never-give-up attitude, you can take control of those feelings and overcome them. Contemplating building a family can be exciting, but always remember that true happiness, peace, joy, and love are not external. They are internal. Start each day with purpose, and decide that you will focus on the blessings that already exist in your life, regardless of what may occur.

It is my prayer that every person who is battling the negative emotional stigmas of infertility is set free and made whole. Life has many wonderful things in store for you. Look forward to each of them so that you can move ahead in abundant love and joy.

Wishing you all the best. Be encouraged and be blessed.

Made in the USA
Coppell, TX
02 April 2021